POTS, MCAS, AND EDS IN ADOLESCENTS

Evidence-Based Guidance for Parents, Teens, and Healthcare Teams Navigating the Trifecta Through the School Years

James Yarrow McGowan

Disclaimer

This book is intended for educational and informational purposes only and does not constitute medical advice, diagnosis, or treatment. The information provided reflects current research and clinical consensus as of the publication date, but medicine changes and new findings may alter recommendations after printing. Always consult a qualified healthcare provider before making decisions about your or your child's medical care. The authors and publisher disclaim all liability for any adverse effects, injury, loss, or damage arising directly or indirectly from the use or application of any information contained in this book. Nothing in this book should be construed as a substitute for professional medical, legal, educational, or psychological services.

All names, identifying details, and personal circumstances used in case examples throughout this book are fictitious. Characters are composites created for illustrative purposes and do not represent any specific individual, living or deceased. Any resemblance to actual persons is entirely coincidental and unintended. No case example should be interpreted as describing a real patient, family, student, or healthcare provider.

The mention of specific medications, treatments, products, organizations, websites, or service providers does not constitute endorsement, recommendation, or guarantee of efficacy or safety by the author or publisher. Medication information is provided for educational reference only and should not be used to self-prescribe, adjust doses, or discontinue treatment without the supervision of a licensed healthcare professional. Treatment decisions must always be made in consultation with the patient's own medical team.

Legal and educational information, including content about Section 504 plans, Individualized Education Programs, disability rights, insurance, and government benefits, reflects federal law as of the publication date and may vary by state, school district, and individual circumstance. This information does not constitute legal advice. Consult a qualified education attorney or disability rights advocate for guidance specific to your situation.

First Edition:2026
ISBN: 978-1-7645936-1-8

Table of Contents

Dedication 1

Preface 2

A Letter to Parents 5

A Letter to Teens 7

How to Use This Handbook 8

PART I UNDERSTANDING THE TRIFECTA IN YOUR TEEN **10**

Chapter 1 Know What Your Teen Faces 11

Chapter 2 Get the Right Diagnosis Faster 18

Chapter 3 Spot the Neurodivergence Overlap 24

PART II MEDICAL MANAGEMENT FOR ADOLESCENTS .. **29**

Chapter 4 Control POTS Symptoms First 30

Chapter 5 Protect Joints in Growing Bodies 34

Chapter 6 Calm the Mast Cell Storm 39

Chapter 7 Make All Three Work Together 44

PART III CONQUERING SCHOOL WITH THE TRIFECTA . **50**

Chapter 8 Claim Your Legal Protections 51

Chapter 9 Get Accommodations That Work 58

Chapter 10 Partner with the School Nurse 66

Chapter 11 Succeed on Tests and Get Into College 73

PART IV THE TEEN EXPERIENCE **80**

Chapter 12 Your Body Is Telling the Truth 81

Chapter 13 Keep Your Social Life Alive 89

Chapter 14 Find What Lights You Up 95

PART V TRANSITIONING TO ADULT CARE **101**

Chapter 15 Start the Transition Early 102

Chapter 16 Find Providers Who Listen 109
Chapter 17 Handle the Legal and Financial Shift 116
Chapter 18 Build a Life That Works 123
PART VI FOR THE PROFESSIONALS 130
Chapter 19 Recognize and Support Trifecta Students 131
Chapter 20 Screen Treat and Transition Together 138
APPENDICES 144
Appendix A Condition Specific Accommodations Checklists 145
Appendix B Templates and Forms 149
Appendix C Medication Quick Reference 155
Appendix D Resources 159
Appendix E Glossary of Medical Terms 162
About the Author 166
References 167

Dedication

To every teen who has been told "it is all in your head" and every parent who knew better.

To the school nurses who stayed late to research a condition they had never heard of.

To the pediatricians who listened when the labs came back normal but the child was clearly suffering.

And to the teenagers reading this right now, sitting in a classroom or lying in bed, wondering if anyone will ever figure out what is wrong: We see you. Your body is real. Your symptoms are real. And this book was written for you.

Preface

Roughly one in every 100 teenagers has postural orthostatic tachycardia syndrome. A significant number of those same teenagers also have hypermobile Ehlers-Danlos syndrome. And a striking percentage of adolescents with both conditions meet the criteria for mast cell activation syndrome. Research shows that the odds of having MCAS are more than 32 times higher in patients who already carry diagnoses of POTS and EDS, a clustering so consistent that clinicians and families have given it a name: the trifecta.

Yet until now, no single resource has addressed these three conditions together in the population where they most commonly appear and cause the most disruption: teenagers.

The medical literature on POTS is growing but remains heavily skewed toward adult populations. Pharmacological treatment guidelines for pediatric POTS are sparse, and most evidence is extrapolated from adult studies. The diagnostic criteria for MCAS are rarely fulfilled in children using standard adult protocols, and many pediatricians have never encountered the diagnosis. EDS research has historically focused on the rarer, more severe subtypes while the most common form, hypermobile EDS, went decades without even a confirmed genetic marker. The result is a generation of adolescents whose conditions are individually under-recognized and collectively unaddressed.

Meanwhile, these teenagers are sitting in classrooms. They are standing in hallways where blood pools in their legs and the room goes gray. They are carrying backpacks that dislocate their shoulders. They are eating cafeteria food that sends their mast cells into overdrive. They are being told by well-meaning adults that they are stressed, anxious, dramatic, or simply going through puberty. And their parents are staying up past midnight, searching medical databases and online forums, trying to assemble a coherent picture from scattered fragments of information.

The families dealing with the trifecta have already tried everything they can find. They have read the dysautonomia pamphlets, joined the EDS support groups, scoured the MCAS websites, and printed stacks of research articles to bring to appointments. What they have not been able to find is a single book that connects all three conditions in the specific context of adolescent life, where school attendance policies, PE requirements, 504 plans, college admissions, and the developmental tasks of identity formation, social connection, and growing independence all collide with a body that does not cooperate.

That is the gap this handbook fills. It is not a medical textbook. It is not a collection of personal stories. It is a practical, evidence-based guide built for the specific challenges that trifecta families face from diagnosis through the transition to adult care. Every chapter ties medical information to actionable next steps. Every accommodation template is designed for the conditions it addresses, not borrowed from a generic disability checklist. Every treatment discussion accounts for the ways these three conditions interact, conflict, and compound each other inside a growing teenage body.

The medical chapters explain each condition in language that families can understand and share with school staff, while maintaining the clinical precision that healthcare providers expect. The school chapters provide legal frameworks, ready-to-use templates, and the specific accommodation language that turns a well-intentioned 504 meeting into a plan that actually works in a hallway, a gymnasium, and a testing room. The teen chapters speak directly to the young person living inside the trifecta, addressing the social, emotional, and identity questions that medical resources rarely touch. And the professional chapters offer school nurses and pediatric teams the screening tools, protocols, and transition strategies that their training did not include.

The trifecta is not three separate problems. It is one interconnected system that demands an interconnected response. The families, schools, and medical teams who understand this principle will produce better outcomes than those who continue treating each condition in isolation.

That principle runs through every page of this handbook, and it is the reason the book was written.

A Letter to Parents

Dear Parent,

I know what brought you here.

Maybe your daughter fainted at school last Tuesday and nobody could explain why. Maybe your son's joints have been aching for two years and four doctors have told you he is fine. Maybe your teenager's skin flushes and swells without warning, and the allergist shrugged and said it was just hives. Maybe you have heard the words POTS, EDS, or MCAS for the first time this week, and you are searching for anything that makes sense.

Or maybe you have known these acronyms for months, even years, and you are exhausted. You have been the researcher, the advocate, the insurance fighter, the school negotiator, and the late-night comforter all at once. You have watched your child lose friends, miss classes, and grieve a version of teenage life that slipped away before they could hold it.

This book was written because no parent should have to piece together a plan from Reddit threads, Facebook groups, and scattered medical articles printed at 2 a.m. You deserve a single resource that explains these three conditions clearly, shows you how they interact in your teenager's body, and gives you concrete tools for school, medical appointments, and the years ahead.

You will find medical information written in plain language, not simplified or dumbed down, but translated with care so that you can understand your child's conditions deeply enough to advocate with confidence. You will find templates you can hand to a school nurse tomorrow morning. You will find chapters written directly to your teen, so they can read the parts that speak to them without needing you to filter everything first.

Most importantly, you will find honesty. This book will not promise a cure. It will not pretend that three pills and a positive attitude will solve everything. But it will show you, clearly and practically, how to help your teen build a life that works with these conditions rather than being defeated by them.

You are already doing the hardest job. This book is here to make it a little less lonely.

With respect and hope,

James Yarrow McGowan

A Letter to Teens

Hey.

I am glad you picked this up. Or maybe your parent handed it to you and you are reading this out of curiosity, or boredom, or because you are stuck in bed again and there is nothing good on your phone. Any reason works.

Here is what I want you to know right away: this book believes you.

If you have been told you are faking it, exaggerating, or just anxious, this book disagrees. If you have been told that everyone gets tired, that dizziness is normal, that your joints are fine because the X-ray looked clean, this book knows better.

POTS, EDS, and MCAS are real medical conditions with real biological causes. They are not in your head. They are not because you are weak. They are not your fault.

Some parts of this book are written for your parents and your medical team. That is because they need tools and information to support you. But several chapters are written directly to you. They cover friendships, dating, school survival, sports grief, social media, and the strange experience of looking perfectly healthy while feeling terrible inside.

You do not have to read this book front to back. Skip to whatever matters most to you right now. Dog-ear the pages. Highlight the parts that feel true. Hand it to a teacher or a friend if you want them to understand.

One more thing. Having these conditions does not define you. They are part of your story, but they are not the whole story. You are still becoming who you are going to be. And that person can be remarkable.

Hang in there. We have a lot of ground to cover.

James Yarrow McGowan

How to Use This Handbook

This book is designed to be used, not just read. It is organized so you can find what you need quickly, whether you are a parent preparing for a school meeting tomorrow, a teen looking for ways to explain your condition to friends, or a school nurse trying to understand a student's emergency protocol.

Finding What You Need

If your teen was just diagnosed, start with Chapters 1 and 2.

If you need school accommodations now, go directly to Chapters 8 and 9.

If your teen is struggling emotionally, Chapter 12 was written for them.

If you are preparing to transition to adult care, Part V gives you a step-by-step timeline.

If you are a school nurse or counselor, Chapters 10 and 19 were written specifically for you.

Worksheets and Templates

This book contains worksheets, templates, and quick-reference cards. You will find them embedded within the relevant chapters and compiled together in Appendix B. Digital versions are available for download at the publisher's website.

A Note on Medical Information

The medical information in this book reflects current research and clinical consensus as of the publication date. Medicine changes. New treatments emerge. Diagnostic criteria evolve. Always confirm treatment decisions with your teen's healthcare providers, and check the publisher's website for updated resource lists.

PART I UNDERSTANDING THE TRIFECTA IN YOUR TEEN

Chapter 1 Know What Your Teen Faces

Clara was fourteen when her body stopped cooperating.

It started with morning dizziness that her mother chalked up to skipping breakfast. Then came the fatigue, so heavy that Clara would fall asleep during third-period English with her head on her desk. Her heart hammered when she stood up from her chair, and sometimes the room went gray around the edges. She dropped out of soccer. Her grades slipped. She stopped texting her friends back because she did not have the energy to be interesting.

Her pediatrician ran blood tests. Everything came back normal. He suggested she might be stressed about school. A second doctor thought she was anemic, but the numbers did not support it. A third wondered about anxiety and prescribed a low dose of sertraline. Clara tried it for six weeks and felt worse.

It was Clara's mother who found the word POTS in an online forum at midnight. She printed three articles, brought them to the next appointment, and asked for a referral to a pediatric cardiologist. The tilt table test confirmed what Clara's body had been screaming for eleven months: her heart rate jumped 52 beats per minute when she stood up. Her autonomic nervous system was not regulating properly.

But the diagnosis did not stop there. The cardiologist noticed Clara's unusually flexible fingers and asked about joint pain. A geneticist confirmed hypermobile Ehlers-Danlos syndrome. And when Clara kept having unexplained flushing, hives, and stomach cramping that no food allergy could explain, an immunologist identified mast cell activation syndrome.

Three conditions. One teenager. Eleven months of being told nothing was wrong.

Clara's story is not unusual. It is, in fact, painfully common. POTS, EDS, and MCAS frequently travel together, forming what clinicians and patients have come to call "the trifecta." Each condition can cause suffering on its own. Together, they create a cascading pattern that can overtake an adolescent's school life, social world, and sense of self.

This chapter will give you and your teen a clear, honest understanding of what each condition is, how it works in a teenage body, and why these three conditions so often appear together.

POTS in Plain Language

Postural orthostatic tachycardia syndrome is a disorder of the autonomic nervous system, the body's autopilot. The autonomic nervous system manages everything your body does without conscious thought: heart rate, blood pressure, digestion, temperature regulation, and the constriction of blood vessels when you stand up.

In a healthy body, standing triggers a rapid series of adjustments. Blood vessels in the lower body tighten to push blood upward. Heart rate adjusts slightly. Blood pressure stays stable. The brain continues to receive adequate blood flow, and you feel nothing unusual.

In a teenager with POTS, this system misfires. When they stand, blood pools in the legs and abdomen. The heart races to compensate, often increasing by 40 or more beats per minute within ten minutes. The brain receives less blood, and the result is dizziness, lightheadedness, tunnel vision, brain fog, nausea, and sometimes fainting.

POTS in adolescents requires a heart rate increase of at least 40 beats per minute upon standing (compared to 30 bpm in adults), the absence of a significant blood pressure drop, and symptoms lasting at least three to six months (Sheldon et al., 2015; Boris & Moak, 2022). The standing heart rate often exceeds 120 beats per minute.

Roughly one in every 100 teenagers is affected (Dysautonomia International, 2023). Onset typically occurs between ages 12 and 15, and more than 75% of adolescent cases occur in females (Boris & Bernadzikowski, 2018). More than half of cases are preceded by an acute viral illness, including COVID-19.

Three broad subtypes are recognized in adolescents, though overlap is common. The neuropathic subtype involves damage to small nerve fibers that control blood vessel constriction. The hyperadrenergic subtype involves excessive norepinephrine release, leading to tremor, anxiety-like symptoms, and elevated blood pressure on standing. The hypovolemic subtype involves low blood volume, which worsens the pooling problem. Many teens show features of more than one subtype.

What makes POTS particularly disruptive in adolescence is its collision with school structure. Teens must stand in hallways, sit upright for hours, climb stairs between classes, and perform in physical education, all activities that directly challenge a dysregulated autonomic system.

EDS in Plain Language

Ehlers-Danlos syndrome is a group of inherited disorders that affect connective tissue, the biological glue that gives structure and support to skin, joints, blood vessels, and internal organs. There are 13 recognized types of EDS, but the type most commonly associated with the trifecta is hypermobile EDS (hEDS) and the closely related hypermobility spectrum disorders (HSD).

Connective tissue in hEDS is too stretchy. Joints bend further than they should, leading to frequent subluxations (partial dislocations), full dislocations, sprains, and chronic joint pain. Skin may be unusually soft, stretchy, or prone to bruising. Wound healing can be slow. Internal organs supported by connective tissue, including blood vessels and the gastrointestinal tract, may also be affected.

The Beighton score is a simple clinical tool used to assess joint hypermobility. It measures flexibility at nine points across the body: the fifth fingers, thumbs, elbows, knees, and spine. A score of 5 out of 9 or higher in adolescents generally suggests generalized hypermobility, though the full diagnostic criteria for hEDS involve additional systemic features and family history (Malfait et al., 2017).

Puberty makes everything harder. Growth spurts destabilize joints that were already too loose. Hormonal fluctuations, particularly estrogen, further affect connective tissue laxity. Menstrual cycles can bring increased pain, heavier bleeding, and worsened joint instability. Many teens with EDS report that their symptoms worsened significantly between ages 11 and 16.

The genetic inheritance conversation matters. Most forms of hEDS follow an autosomal dominant pattern, meaning a child has a 50% chance of inheriting the condition from an affected parent. Many parents discover their own EDS only after their child is diagnosed.

For families, the hardest part of EDS is often its invisibility. A teen with hEDS does not look injured. Their joints do not appear swollen. Their X-rays and MRIs often look normal. And because the condition is genetic, they have never known a body that works differently. They may not realize that the pain they feel is not what everyone feels.

MCAS in Plain Language

Mast cell activation syndrome is a condition in which mast cells, a type of immune cell found in nearly every tissue in the body, become overactive and release their chemical contents inappropriately.

Mast cells are normally helpful. They detect threats like bacteria, parasites, and allergens, and they release chemicals (mediators) including histamine, prostaglandins, leukotrienes, and tryptase to mount an immune response. In a healthy system, this process is tightly controlled.

In MCAS, the system loses control. Mast cells release their mediators too easily, too often, and in response to triggers that should not provoke a reaction: temperature changes, fragrances, stress, certain foods, vibration, sunlight, exercise, or even standing up.

The resulting symptoms can affect nearly every organ system. Skin symptoms include flushing, hives, itching, and swelling. Gastrointestinal symptoms include nausea, cramping, diarrhea, and food intolerances that shift unpredictably. Cardiovascular symptoms include rapid heart rate and low blood pressure. Neurological symptoms include brain fog, headaches, and dizziness. In severe cases, mast cell activation can trigger anaphylaxis, a medical emergency requiring epinephrine.

Diagnosing MCAS in adolescents is particularly challenging. The formal diagnostic criteria require clinical symptoms affecting two or more organ systems, evidence of elevated mast cell mediators (typically measured through blood tryptase levels or 24-hour urine collections for histamine metabolites and prostaglandins), and improvement with mast cell-targeted medications (Valent et al., 2019). But mast cell mediator levels fluctuate, are difficult to capture during flares, and may not rise high enough in children to meet adult thresholds (Australasian Mastocytosis Society, 2026).

Many pediatricians have never heard of MCAS. When they encounter a teenager with recurrent flushing, unexplained GI distress, and allergic-type reactions without identifiable allergens, the diagnosis is often missed or attributed to anxiety, attention seeking, or food sensitivity.

The hereditary alpha tryptasemia (HaT) genetic trait, present in 4% to 6% of White populations, is associated with elevated baseline tryptase and multi-system symptoms that overlap significantly with MCAS, including POTS-like symptoms (Castells et al., 2024). Testing for HaT is becoming more available and may help clarify the picture for some families.

How the Three Conditions Feed Each Other

Understanding each condition separately is only the first step. The real challenge of the trifecta is understanding how POTS, EDS, and MCAS interact, amplify each other, and create a cycle that no single treatment can break alone.

Think of it this way. EDS affects the scaffolding of the body. When connective tissue is too stretchy, blood vessels are too flexible to constrict properly when your teen stands up. Blood pools. The heart races. POTS symptoms appear.

POTS affects the wiring. When the autonomic nervous system misfires, it disrupts digestion, temperature regulation, and blood flow to every organ, including the gut, where a large concentration of mast cells live.

MCAS affects the security system. When mast cells overreact, they release histamine and other inflammatory chemicals that damage connective tissue, worsen blood vessel instability, increase gut inflammation, and directly trigger autonomic dysfunction.

The result is a self-perpetuating cycle. Gut dysfunction from MCAS and dysautonomia leads to poor nutrient absorption. Poor nutrition weakens collagen production. Weakened collagen worsens joint instability and vascular laxity. Vascular laxity worsens POTS. POTS flares trigger stress responses that activate mast cells. And the cycle continues.

Research confirms this clustering. In one study, 31% of patients with both POTS and EDS also met criteria for MCAS, compared to only 2% of patients without POTS or EDS (Cheung & Vadas, 2015). The odds ratio was 32.46, an extraordinarily strong association. Another study found mast cell mediator abnormalities in 42% of POTS patients who also had allergic and gastrointestinal symptoms (Shibao et al., 2005).

Some researchers now describe an expanded pattern called the Pentad, which adds autoimmune disorders and gastrointestinal dysfunction to the trifecta. This broader framework reflects the clinical reality that many teens with POTS, EDS, and MCAS also develop autoimmune thyroid disease, celiac disease, or severe gastroparesis over time.

For parents, the most important takeaway is this: if your teen has been diagnosed with one of these conditions and still has unexplained symptoms, push for evaluation of the other two. Treating POTS alone while ignoring underlying MCAS will produce limited results. Stabilizing joints with physical therapy while missing the autonomic dysfunction that keeps your teen bedridden will not restore their school attendance. The trifecta demands a trifecta response.

Action Step: Draw a simple triangle on a piece of paper with your teen. Label each corner with one condition: POTS, EDS, MCAS. In the center, write the symptoms your teen experiences. Draw lines connecting each symptom to the condition or conditions that might be driving it. This is your family's first trifecta map, and it will help you communicate with every provider you see.

In a Nutshell

POTS disrupts your teen's autonomic nervous system, making standing, concentrating, and physical activity unreliable. In adolescents, the diagnostic threshold is a heart rate increase of 40 bpm or more upon standing.

EDS weakens the connective tissue that holds your teen's body together, causing joint instability, chronic pain, and vascular problems that worsen during the growth and hormonal changes of puberty.

MCAS causes your teen's mast cells to overreact, releasing inflammatory chemicals in response to triggers that should be harmless, creating symptoms across skin, gut, cardiovascular, and neurological systems.

These three conditions cluster together with striking frequency. Treating one while ignoring the others rarely produces lasting improvement. The trifecta demands that families, schools, and healthcare teams understand all three conditions and address them as an interconnected system.

Your teen's body is not broken. It is wired differently. And once you understand the wiring, you can start working with it instead of against it.

Chapter 2 Get the Right Diagnosis Faster

Hugo was twelve when he started getting headaches that lasted for days. His mother, a middle school teacher, assumed he needed glasses. The optometrist said his vision was fine. Over the next four months, Hugo added dizziness to the headaches, then nausea, then episodes where his heart felt like it was trying to escape his chest. He stopped playing basketball. He started missing Mondays.

His pediatrician ordered basic blood work: complete blood count, thyroid panel, metabolic panel. All normal. A neurologist ran an EEG and an MRI. Both clean. Hugo was told he was probably stressed about seventh grade.

His mother was not convinced. She noticed that Hugo's symptoms were worse in the morning, worse when standing in line for lunch, and worse on hot days. She started recording his heart rate with a phone app. Lying down: 68. Standing for five minutes: 124. Standing for ten minutes: 131. She brought the data to the next appointment.

The pediatrician looked at the numbers, paused, and said, "I think we need to send him to cardiology."

It took Hugo fourteen months from first symptom to diagnosis. Research suggests this is typical. Families of adolescents with POTS report visiting an average of seven healthcare providers before receiving an accurate diagnosis (Shaw et al., 2019). For EDS, the diagnostic delay averages over a decade in adult populations, though awareness is slowly improving for younger patients. MCAS, the newest of the three diagnoses, often takes even longer because many physicians have not yet learned to screen for it.

The diagnostic process does not have to take this long. This chapter will teach you what red flags to watch for, which specialists to seek, what tests to request, and how to advocate effectively when the medical system moves too slowly or does not listen.

Red Flags That Deserve Investigation

Certain symptom patterns in teenagers should raise concern, even when initial lab work returns normal. Normal labs do not mean a normal body. They mean the tests that were ordered did not find anything. The right tests may not have been ordered yet.

Watch for fatigue that does not improve with sleep. Teenagers are often tired, but a teen with POTS or MCAS describes fatigue that rest does not touch. They wake up exhausted. They need hours to feel functional. Naps do not restore them.

Watch for recurrent dizziness or fainting, particularly in the morning, during prolonged standing, after hot showers, or in warm environments. This is not "growing too fast" or "forgetting to eat breakfast." This is orthostatic intolerance, and it demands evaluation.

Watch for unexplained rashes, flushing, hives, or allergic-type reactions that appear without a clear allergen. When allergy testing returns negative but the reactions continue, MCAS should be considered.

Watch for joint pain that comes and goes, affects multiple joints, and does not correspond to a specific injury. If your teen is called "double-jointed" and also reports pain, the combination points toward hypermobility that may warrant formal evaluation.

Watch for chronic gastrointestinal symptoms: nausea, abdominal pain, bloating, diarrhea, constipation, or food intolerances that seem to shift. The gut is heavily innervated by the autonomic nervous system and densely populated with mast cells. GI dysfunction is a common overlap point for all three conditions.

Watch for "brain fog," the inability to concentrate, recall information, or process language quickly, particularly when it fluctuates with posture, hydration, or time of day. This is not laziness. It is reduced cerebral blood flow, and it has a name.

Action Step: Before your next medical appointment, keep a two-week symptom diary. Record the time of day, activity, posture, and severity of each symptom on a 1 to 10 scale. Note heart rate upon waking and after standing for five and ten minutes. Patterns in this data can shift a conversation from "your teen seems fine" to "we need further evaluation."

Building the Right Diagnostic Team

The trifecta spans multiple medical specialties, and no single doctor can diagnose and manage all three conditions alone. Knowing which specialists to seek, and in what order, prevents months of circular referrals.

Start with a pediatric cardiologist for POTS evaluation. Pediatric cardiologists are more familiar with the adolescent diagnostic criteria (40 bpm threshold) and more experienced with tilt table testing in younger patients. An adult cardiologist may not recognize the presentation or may apply the wrong diagnostic threshold.

For EDS evaluation, a medical geneticist is the gold standard. Geneticists are trained in the formal diagnostic criteria for all 13 types of EDS and can distinguish hEDS from other connective tissue disorders. A rheumatologist can also evaluate hypermobility, but some rheumatologists are unfamiliar with the 2017 hEDS criteria. If you go the rheumatology route, confirm before scheduling that the provider has experience with EDS in adolescents.

For MCAS workup, seek an allergist/immunologist with specific experience in mast cell disorders. General allergists may focus exclusively on IgE-mediated allergies and miss non-allergic mast cell activation. The Mast Cell Disease Society maintains a provider directory that can help locate experienced clinicians.

Above all, identify a coordinating primary care provider who is willing to learn, communicate across specialties, and serve as the "quarterback" for your teen's care. This may be your pediatrician, a family medicine physician, or an adolescent medicine specialist. The coordinator does not need to know everything about the trifecta. They need to be willing to listen, read, and connect the pieces.

Diagnostic Testing Demystified

The tilt table test is the primary diagnostic tool for POTS. Your teen lies flat on a motorized table while heart rate and blood pressure are monitored. After a period of rest, the table tilts to a near-upright position (60 to 70 degrees). If the heart rate increases by 40 or more beats per minute (in adolescents) within ten minutes without a significant drop in blood pressure, and your teen experiences symptoms of orthostatic intolerance, the test supports a POTS diagnosis.

Preparation matters. Your teen should be well-hydrated before the test. Medications that affect heart rate (beta-blockers, stimulants) may need to be paused per the ordering physician's instructions. The test can provoke symptoms including dizziness, nausea, and fainting. Know that this is expected and temporary.

If a tilt table test is not available, the active standing test is a reliable alternative. Your teen lies flat for five minutes while heart rate and blood pressure are recorded. They then stand motionless for ten minutes while measurements are taken at one-minute intervals. The same diagnostic criteria apply.

For EDS, the Beighton score and a comprehensive clinical evaluation are the primary tools. There is no blood test for hEDS. Genetic testing can confirm several other types of EDS (classical, vascular, kyphoscoliotic), but the gene responsible for hEDS has not yet been identified. Diagnosis is clinical, based on joint hypermobility, systemic features (soft skin, easy bruising, GI dysfunction, chronic pain), and family history.

For MCAS, the laboratory workup centers on measuring mast cell mediators during symptomatic episodes. Serum tryptase drawn within four hours of a flare is the most commonly ordered test, though many MCAS patients have normal baseline tryptase levels. Twenty-four-hour urine collections for N-methylhistamine, prostaglandin D2 metabolites, and leukotriene E4 may be more revealing. Timing is everything. Testing during a quiet period will often miss the elevations. Testing during or immediately after a flare is far more likely to capture abnormal levels.

When the System Fails You

Eloise's mother knew something was wrong for three years before any doctor agreed. Eloise was nine when the joint pain started, eleven when the fainting began, and twelve when an emergency room physician told her mother, in front of Eloise, that "some children learn that being sick gets them out of school."

This kind of dismissal happens too often. It happens because these conditions are poorly covered in medical training. It happens because the primary symptoms, pain, fatigue, dizziness, and nausea, overlap with anxiety and depression. It happens because teenage girls are disproportionately disbelieved by the medical system.

If your teen's concerns are being dismissed, here are concrete steps you can take.

Document everything. Keep a written log of symptoms, appointments, and what each provider said. Take photos of visible symptoms (rashes, joint hyperextension, flushing episodes). Record heart rate data using a phone app or fitness tracker. This creates an evidence base that is harder to dismiss than a verbal description.

Use specific language when requesting tests. Instead of "I think something is wrong," say "I am requesting a tilt table test to evaluate for postural orthostatic tachycardia syndrome. My daughter's standing heart rate consistently exceeds 120 bpm, and she meets the screening criteria based on her symptom pattern." Specificity signals that you have done your research and know what you are asking for.

Request that refusals be documented. If a provider declines to order a test or referral, ask them to note in the medical record that you requested it and that they declined. This single sentence changes the dynamic of the conversation.

Seek a second opinion without guilt. You are not being difficult. You are being thorough. A second opinion is a standard and respected part of medical care.

Action Step: Prepare a one-page medical summary for every new specialist appointment. Include: your teen's diagnoses (confirmed and suspected), current medications, key lab results, a brief symptom timeline, and the specific question you want this specialist to answer. This saves time, prevents miscommunication, and demonstrates that you are an organized and informed advocate.

In a Nutshell

The diagnostic process for the trifecta is often slower than it should be. Adolescents wait an average of one to two years for a POTS diagnosis alone, and longer when EDS and MCAS are also present.

Red flags that warrant further investigation include fatigue unrelieved by rest, recurrent dizziness upon standing, unexplained allergic-type reactions, multi-joint pain, chronic GI distress, and fluctuating brain fog.

The right diagnostic team includes a pediatric cardiologist for POTS, a medical geneticist for EDS, an allergist/immunologist for MCAS, and a coordinating primary care provider willing to connect the pieces.

When the system fails you, documentation, specific language, recorded refusals, and second opinions are your strongest tools.

You know your child. Trust that knowledge. And do not stop advocating until the tests match what your eyes can see.

Chapter 3 Spot the Neurodivergence Overlap

Felix had been managing his POTS with salt tablets and compression stockings for a year when his mother made an observation that changed everything. "He cannot remember to take his medications," she told the cardiologist, "even when they are sitting right next to his water bottle. He cannot organize his backpack. He loses his symptom journal every week. I do not think this is just brain fog."

She was right. Neuropsychological testing revealed that Felix had ADHD, primarily inattentive type. The executive function challenges that his family had attributed entirely to POTS were, in part, a separate neurodevelopmental condition that had been there all along, masked by years of compensatory effort and then unmasked by the exhaustion of chronic illness.

Felix is not an outlier. Emerging research shows striking overlap between EDS and neurodivergence. People with EDS are approximately 7.5 times more likely to be autistic and 5.5 times more likely to have ADHD than the general population (Casanova et al., 2020; Cederlof et al., 2016). Studies suggest that between 32% and 74% of people with ADHD may have hypermobility, and between 13% and 53% of autistic people may have EDS, though actual rates are likely higher because both populations are systematically underdiagnosed (Eccles et al., 2021).

This is not a coincidence. Connective tissue is not limited to joints and skin. It provides the structural framework for the nervous system itself. When connective tissue is atypical, the nervous system develops atypically. The same genetic variations that produce hypermobile joints may also produce different patterns of sensory processing, executive function, and social cognition.

For families managing the trifecta, this overlap matters enormously. A teen with POTS, EDS, MCAS, and unidentified ADHD will struggle to follow complex medication schedules, remember to hydrate, advocate with teachers, and organize the paperwork that school accommodations require. A teen with the trifecta and unidentified autism may have difficulty interpreting body signals (a skill called interoception), tolerating the sensory load of MCAS triggers, and communicating needs to medical providers in ways that providers expect.

If neurodivergence is not identified, parents and providers may blame the teen for "not trying hard enough" to manage their conditions, when in reality, the management strategies being offered do not match how their brain works.

When Executive Function and Chronic Illness Collide

Executive function is the set of mental skills that allow a person to plan, organize, prioritize, remember instructions, manage time, and regulate behavior. ADHD impairs executive function. POTS impairs executive function. Together, they create a double deficit that can make even simple daily health tasks feel overwhelming.

Consider what trifecta management requires of a teenager: tracking symptoms daily, remembering multiple medications at specific times, drinking measured amounts of fluid, eating low-histamine foods prepared in specific ways, wearing compression garments, performing prescribed exercise, communicating with teachers about accommodations, and attending appointments with multiple specialists. This is a project management load that many healthy adults would find demanding.

For a teen with ADHD, these tasks may require external scaffolding: pill organizers, phone alarms, visual checklists, simplified routines, and parent involvement that goes beyond what their peers require. Without this scaffolding, the teen may appear noncompliant with treatment when they are actually struggling with a neurological barrier to compliance.

Action Step: If your teen has been diagnosed with the trifecta and struggles to follow their management plan despite motivation and effort, request a neuropsychological evaluation that specifically assesses executive function, working memory, and processing speed. Share the results with your teen's medical team so treatment plans can be adapted to match how your teen's brain actually works.

Sensory Processing and MCAS Triggers

Many neurodivergent teens experience sensory processing differences. Sounds may be too loud. Textures may be unbearable. Lights may be too bright. Smells may be overpowering. For a teen who is also managing MCAS, sensory sensitivities and mast cell triggers can overlap in ways that are difficult to distinguish.

Is the fluorescent lighting causing a migraine because of sensory sensitivity, or because it triggered a mast cell response? Is the food aversion driven by autism-related texture sensitivity, MCAS-related food reactivity, or both? Is the school cafeteria intolerable because of the noise, the smells, or the invisible chemical exposures?

In practice, the answer is often "all of the above." Sensory processing differences and mast cell activation may share underlying neurobiological pathways. The clinical implication is that environmental modifications, reducing sensory load, controlling temperature, minimizing chemical exposures, and providing quiet spaces, can help both conditions simultaneously.

Interoception and Body Signal Confusion

Interoception is the ability to perceive and interpret internal body signals: hunger, thirst, pain, heart rate, temperature, and the need to use the bathroom. Research shows that many autistic people and people with ADHD have atypical interoception (Garfinkel et al., 2016). They may not notice hunger until they are shaking. They may not notice pain until it is severe. They may not notice rising heart rate until they are about to faint.

For a teen with POTS, accurate interoception can be the difference between sitting down before a faint and hitting the floor. For a teen with MCAS, recognizing the early signs of a mast cell flare (warmth, flushing, itching) can mean the difference between taking rescue medication early and ending up in the emergency room.

When a teen has both atypical interoception and the trifecta, they need external monitoring tools to supplement what their body is not accurately reporting. Heart rate watches, hydration tracking apps, scheduled medication alarms, and visual body check-in systems can fill the gaps that impaired interoception creates.

Getting the Full Picture

Zoe's parents spent three years focused entirely on her POTS, EDS, and MCAS diagnoses before a school psychologist noticed that Zoe also met criteria for autism. Looking back, the signs had been there all along: intense special interests, difficulty with unstructured social situations, preference for sameness and routine, and overwhelm in loud or crowded environments. But every autistic trait had been attributed to chronic illness. "Of course she avoids the cafeteria. She has MCAS." "Of course she prefers routine. Her symptoms are unpredictable." "Of course she has trouble with friends. She misses school all the time."

Each of these explanations was partially true. But they were incomplete. And without understanding the autism, Zoe's support plan was missing a fundamental layer.

If your teen has the trifecta and you recognize patterns that go beyond what the medical conditions explain, bring your observations to a provider who understands both chronic illness and neurodevelopmental differences. Neuropsychologists, developmental pediatricians, and psychologists who specialize in autism assessment can evaluate your teen in the context of their medical conditions, rather than attributing everything to illness or dismissing everything as "behavioral."

Action Step: Write down three to five observations about your teen that you have noticed but have not been able to fully explain through the trifecta diagnoses alone. Bring this list to a provider who can help determine whether further neurodevelopmental screening is warranted.

In a Nutshell

The overlap between EDS and neurodivergence (autism and ADHD) is far more common than previously understood. Teens with the trifecta who also have unidentified neurodivergence may appear noncompliant with treatment when they are actually facing neurological barriers to self-management.

Executive function challenges from ADHD compound the organizational demands of managing three chronic conditions. Sensory processing differences from autism can overlap with and amplify MCAS triggers. Atypical interoception can impair a teen's ability to recognize early warning signs of POTS episodes or MCAS flares.

Identifying neurodivergence alongside the trifecta allows families and providers to build management plans that work with the teen's brain, not against it. This single insight can transform outcomes for teenagers who have been struggling despite their best efforts.

PART II MEDICAL MANAGEMENT FOR ADOLESCENTS

Chapter 4 Control POTS Symptoms First

Noemi was fifteen and had not attended a full week of school in seven months. Her POTS diagnosis was confirmed, but the general advice she received ("drink more water and eat more salt") was not enough to get her out of bed before noon. Her heart rate reached 140 within three minutes of standing. By the time she made it to her second class, she was so lightheaded that she had to put her head on her desk. By lunch, she was in the nurse's office. By 1 p.m., her mother was picking her up.

The turning point came when Noemi's cardiologist moved beyond general advice and built a structured, layered treatment protocol. Not one single intervention, but a system of non-pharmacological strategies combined with carefully chosen medications, all timed around the school day.

Within six weeks, Noemi was attending school until noon. By three months, she was making it to her last class most days. By six months, she was back to nearly full attendance, with accommodations in place for the hard days.

POTS treatment in adolescents follows a clear hierarchy: non-pharmacological foundations first, medications layered on top when needed, and exercise as the single most effective long-term intervention. No single treatment works alone. The protocol that helps your teen is the one that combines the right strategies in the right sequence for their specific symptoms and school schedule.

Build the Foundation Before Adding Medication

The first-line treatment for adolescent POTS is not a pill. It is a set of daily habits that increase blood volume, improve vascular tone, and reduce the physiological conditions that make standing unbearable.

Fluid intake for a teenager with POTS should be significantly higher than typical recommendations. Most guidelines suggest 2 to 3 liters of non-caffeinated fluid daily, which translates to roughly 64 to 100 ounces (Boris & Moak, 2022). This is not drinking when thirsty. This is drinking on a schedule, before thirst signals appear, because thirst in POTS patients often lags behind actual dehydration.

Sodium supplementation works alongside fluid loading to expand blood volume. Clinical recommendations typically range from 3 to 10 grams of sodium per day for adolescents with POTS, depending on severity and body weight (Raj et al., 2020). Salt tablets, electrolyte drinks, and strategic salty snacks can all contribute. For school, portable electrolyte packets that dissolve in water bottles are practical and discreet.

Compression garments counteract the blood pooling in the lower body that drives POTS symptoms. Waist-high compression stockings (20 to 30 mmHg or 30 to 40 mmHg) are more effective than knee-high styles because they compress the abdominal venous reservoir. The challenge for teenagers is social. Few fifteen-year-olds want to wear medical compression stockings. Abdominal compression bands and compression athletic wear (leggings, shorts) can provide benefit with less visibility.

Sleep hygiene in teens with POTS requires extra attention. Dysautonomia often disrupts circadian rhythms, leading to delayed sleep onset, non-restorative sleep, and severe morning symptoms. A consistent sleep schedule, elimination of screens in the last hour before bed, slight elevation of the head of the bed (4 to 6 inches), and avoidance of large meals or hot baths before sleep can improve overnight autonomic regulation.

When Medication Becomes Necessary

When non-pharmacological strategies alone do not produce adequate symptom control, medications can be added in a targeted, stepwise fashion. Published literature on pharmacological treatment of pediatric POTS is limited compared to adult studies, and treatment decisions should always involve a physician experienced in adolescent dysautonomia (Huynh et al., 2024).

Fludrocortisone is a synthetic mineralocorticoid that promotes sodium and water retention, expanding blood volume. It is often the first medication tried. Side effects can include low potassium, headaches, and swelling, so electrolyte monitoring is important.

Midodrine is a vasoconstrictor that tightens blood vessels and reduces pooling. It works quickly (within an hour) and wears off in about four hours, making timing around the school day critical. A dose before school and at lunchtime can cover the highest-demand hours. Because midodrine raises blood pressure, it should not be taken before lying down.

Beta-blockers like metoprolol and propranolol reduce heart rate but can also cause fatigue, exercise intolerance, and cognitive dulling, side effects that are particularly problematic for students. Low doses may help teens with hyperadrenergic POTS, but the cognitive trade-offs must be weighed against the school demands.

Ivabradine, a newer option, reduces heart rate without lowering blood pressure or causing the cognitive effects associated with beta-blockers. Emerging evidence in pediatric populations is promising, though it is often used off-label and may require insurance authorization (Huynh et al., 2024).

Exercise as the Most Powerful Long-Term Tool

Exercise is the single most studied and most effective treatment for POTS. Regular aerobic exercise increases blood volume, improves cardiac function, enhances vascular tone, and reduces symptom severity over time (Fu et al., 2010). The challenge for teenagers with POTS is that the very thing that will help them most, moving their body, is also what makes them feel worst.

The modified CHOP (Children's Hospital of Philadelphia) protocol addresses this by starting with recumbent exercise that does not require standing: recumbent cycling, rowing, swimming, and floor-based strength exercises. Over weeks and months, the protocol gradually introduces upright activities as the cardiovascular system strengthens.

For school PE departments, this means standard PE expectations need to change. Your teen may need a physician-prescribed exercise plan that replaces traditional PE activities with recumbent alternatives. A recumbent bike in the nurse's office or gym, swimming during a scheduled period, or a documented home exercise log can satisfy PE requirements while protecting your teen from harm.

Action Step: Ask your teen's cardiologist for a written exercise prescription that specifies what types of exercise are safe, what modifications are needed, and what signs should trigger stopping. Give a copy to the school PE teacher and include it in your teen's 504 plan.

In a Nutshell

POTS treatment in adolescents follows a layered approach: non-pharmacological foundations (fluids, sodium, compression, sleep) first, then targeted medications when needed, with structured exercise as the most powerful long-term intervention.

No single intervention works alone. The protocol that restores school attendance is the one that combines the right strategies for your teen's specific subtype, symptom pattern, and school schedule.

Exercise is the strongest evidence-based treatment, but it must start recumbent and progress gradually. Standard PE expectations must be modified, not waived.

Every medication has trade-offs that affect school performance. Discuss cognitive side effects explicitly with your prescriber and time doses around academic demands.

Chapter 5 Protect Joints in Growing Bodies

Mateo dislocated his shoulder for the third time during a basketball game in ninth grade. Each time, the team trainer popped it back in and sent him home with ice. Each time, his parents assumed it was a sports injury that would heal. But when Mateo mentioned that his fingers sometimes "popped out" while holding a pencil, and that his knees buckled going down stairs, his mother started paying closer attention.

A geneticist confirmed hypermobile Ehlers-Danlos syndrome. Looking back, the clues had been everywhere. Mateo had always been the most flexible kid in gym class. He could bend his thumb to his wrist and hyperextend his elbows past straight. His skin bruised easily. He had been told since elementary school that he was "double-jointed," as though it were a party trick.

It was not a party trick. It was a connective tissue disorder that, without proper management, would continue to damage his joints with every unmodified activity.

Managing EDS in a teenager whose body is still growing requires a different approach than managing it in an adult. Growth spurts stretch already-loose ligaments further. Hormonal changes during puberty, particularly rising estrogen, can increase tissue laxity. And the natural risk-taking behavior of adolescence does not mix well with joints that dislocate without warning.

Stability Over Flexibility

The old model of physical therapy, which emphasized stretching and increasing range of motion, can be harmful for teens with EDS. Their joints already move too far. What they need is the opposite: stability.

Modern physical therapy for hypermobile teens focuses on joint stabilization through strengthening the muscles around unstable joints, proprioception training (teaching the body to sense where it is in space), and neuromuscular control exercises that help the muscles react quickly enough to protect joints from sudden movements.

Kinesio taping can provide additional joint support during the school day without restricting movement entirely. Many teens find it less visible and more comfortable than rigid braces. Parents can learn basic taping techniques from their physical therapist, and teens can learn to tape their own most vulnerable joints (fingers, wrists, ankles, and knees).

Bracing has a role but should be used strategically. Rigid braces prevent dislocation but also prevent the muscles from doing their stabilization work. Over time, excessive bracing can lead to further muscle weakening and increased dependence. A physical therapist experienced in EDS should guide decisions about when to brace, for how long, and during which activities.

Pain Without a Quick Fix

Chronic pain is one of the most debilitating features of adolescent EDS, and it does not respond well to the usual approaches. Over-the-counter pain relievers provide limited relief. Opioids are inappropriate for chronic use in teenagers and carry serious risks. The path forward requires a multimodal strategy that addresses pain from several angles simultaneously.

Low-dose naltrexone (LDN), typically prescribed at 1 to 4.5 mg daily, has shown promise for reducing chronic pain and neuroinflammation in connective tissue disorders. It works differently from standard pain medications by modulating the immune system and endorphin pathways rather than blocking pain signals directly. Evidence is still emerging, and not all providers are familiar with it, but families may wish to discuss it with their medical team (Younger et al., 2014).

Topical options, including lidocaine patches, menthol-based creams, and anti-inflammatory gels applied directly to painful joints, can provide localized relief without systemic side effects that affect school performance.

Cognitive behavioral approaches to pain help teens change their relationship with chronic pain rather than eliminating it entirely. Pain neuroscience education teaches teens that pain signals in EDS are often amplified by a sensitized nervous system, not proportional to actual tissue damage. This understanding can reduce fear of movement and improve willingness to engage in stabilization exercises.

Sleep disruption worsens pain, and pain disrupts sleep, creating a cycle that is particularly destructive during adolescence. Addressing sleep quality through sleep hygiene, appropriate sleep positioning (supportive pillows for hypermobile necks and shoulders), and, when necessary, sleep-supporting medications can break this cycle.

Keeping Teens Safe at School and in Sports

School presents specific physical risks for teens with EDS. Heavy backpacks strain unstable shoulders, wrists, and spines. Prolonged sitting in poorly designed chairs causes pain and fatigue. Stairs threaten unstable knees and ankles. Standard PE activities, from dodgeball to rope climbing, can cause injuries that take weeks to heal.

Backpack weight should not exceed 10% to 15% of the teen's body weight. Rolling backpacks, duplicate textbook sets (one at home, one in the classroom), and digital textbooks can reduce the daily load. Locker placement near classrooms reduces carrying distance.

Contact sports carry elevated risk for teens with EDS due to joint instability and, in some EDS types, tissue fragility. The decision to participate in sports should be made individually, with input from the teen's medical team, the teen themselves, and the family. Low-impact activities (swimming, cycling, Pilates, yoga with modifications) are generally safer and can also support the stabilization goals of physical therapy.

Musical instruments require attention too. Wind instruments increase intrathoracic pressure, which can be problematic for some EDS patients. String instruments, particularly violin, place sustained stress on the wrist, shoulder, and neck. Occupational therapy can help adapt technique, and teachers should understand that accommodations may be needed.

Growing Into a Changing Body

Puberty is hard enough without EDS. Growth spurts destabilize joints that were already loose. Long bones grow faster than the surrounding muscles can strengthen, leaving joints temporarily more vulnerable. Many teens with EDS report significant worsening of pain, instability, and subluxations during the growth years of 11 to 16.

For girls with EDS, menstruation adds another layer. Heavy menstrual bleeding is common in connective tissue disorders because the tissue of the uterine lining is more fragile and bleeds more easily. Menstrual pain can be disproportionately severe. Hormonal fluctuations across the menstrual cycle affect connective tissue laxity, with many girls reporting increased subluxations in the days before their period.

These issues deserve direct conversation with the teen's gynecologist or primary care provider. Hormonal management (oral contraceptives, IUDs) may help stabilize both the menstrual symptoms and the cyclical worsening of joint instability.

Action Step: Request a physical therapy evaluation with a provider experienced in hypermobility. Ask specifically for a stabilization-focused program, not a flexibility program. Bring the provider a list of your teen's most frequently injured or painful joints to guide the initial assessment.

In a Nutshell

EDS management in growing teens requires stability over flexibility. Physical therapy should focus on joint stabilization, proprioception, and neuromuscular control, not increasing range of motion.

Pain management demands a multimodal approach: topical options, low-dose naltrexone, cognitive behavioral strategies, and sleep quality improvement. Opioids are not appropriate for chronic adolescent EDS pain.

School safety requires attention to backpack weight, PE modifications, stair navigation, and seating ergonomics. Sports decisions should be individualized with medical input.

Puberty intensifies EDS symptoms through growth spurts, hormonal fluctuations, and menstrual complications. These changes are predictable and manageable with proactive planning.

Chapter 6 Calm the Mast Cell Storm

Lucia was thirteen when she ate a strawberry and her face swelled so severely that her father drove her to the emergency room. The ER doctor gave her epinephrine and told her she had a strawberry allergy. But when the allergist ran a full panel two weeks later, every result came back negative. No IgE-mediated allergies were detected.

Over the next several months, Lucia reacted to strawberries again, but also to heat, perfume, the chlorine in the school pool, the new carpet in her classroom, and on one alarming occasion, to exercise during PE. Each reaction looked different. Sometimes it was hives. Sometimes it was cramping so severe she could not stand. Sometimes her throat felt tight and her heart pounded. Sometimes it was brain fog so dense she could not remember her locker combination.

Her allergist, to his credit, recognized the pattern. "These are not typical allergies," he told Lucia's parents. "These are mast cells that are too reactive." He started her on a layered antihistamine protocol and ordered a 24-hour urine collection during her next flare. Prostaglandin D2 metabolites came back elevated. Lucia had mast cell activation syndrome.

MCAS management in adolescents centers on three strategies: identifying and avoiding triggers, using medications to stabilize mast cells and block their chemical output, and preparing for the possibility that despite best efforts, severe reactions may occur.

Finding and Avoiding Triggers in a Teenager's World

The first challenge of MCAS management is that triggers are individual, inconsistent, and often invisible. A trigger that causes a severe reaction one week may cause nothing the next. A food that was safe for months may suddenly provoke symptoms. This unpredictability is one of the most frustrating aspects of the condition for teenagers, who crave the normalcy and spontaneity of adolescent life.

Common trigger categories include temperature extremes (both hot and cold), physical exertion, emotional stress, strong fragrances (perfumes, cleaning products, candles), certain foods (particularly those high in histamine, such as aged cheeses, fermented foods, cured meats, and leftover proteins), infections, hormonal fluctuations, and some medications (NSAIDs, certain antibiotics, and contrast dye).

The elimination approach starts with removing the most common triggers and establishing a "safe baseline," a set of conditions under which the teen is relatively stable. From there, triggers are reintroduced one at a time to identify individual patterns. This process requires patience, detailed journaling, and the recognition that the goal is not to find every trigger but to identify the most impactful ones.

School environments present specific MCAS challenges. Cafeteria food is often high in histamine. Cleaning chemicals used in classrooms and bathrooms contain volatile organic compounds that can trigger mast cells. Science labs involve chemical exposures. Gymnasiums are hot and poorly ventilated. Art rooms contain solvents and adhesives. Each of these environments may need to be addressed in your teen's accommodation plan.

Medication Protocols That Work Around the School Day

The pharmacological management of MCAS in adolescents typically follows a layered approach, starting with medications that block histamine receptors and adding mast cell stabilizers as needed.

H1 antihistamines (cetirizine, fexofenadine, loratadine) block the histamine that causes itching, flushing, and hives. H2 antihistamines (famotidine, ranitidine alternatives) block histamine in the gastrointestinal tract, helping with nausea, cramping, and acid reflux. Many teens with MCAS take both an H1 and an H2 antihistamine daily as baseline prevention.

Mast cell stabilizers, including cromolyn sodium (taken orally before meals to protect the GI tract) and ketotifen (which also has antihistamine properties), work by preventing mast cells from releasing their contents in the first place. These medications are preventive, not rescue, and must be taken consistently to be effective.

Leukotriene modifiers like montelukast block another category of inflammatory mediators released by mast cells. They can help with respiratory symptoms, nasal congestion, and some skin symptoms.

For teens with severe or refractory MCAS, omalizumab (an anti-IgE monoclonal antibody) may be considered. It is administered by injection and requires specialist oversight.

Timing medications around the school day is a practical challenge that is rarely discussed in clinical settings but matters enormously for teens. A sedating antihistamine taken in the morning will impair concentration during first period. Cromolyn sodium taken 30 minutes before meals requires a level of planning that few middle schoolers can manage independently. Work with your teen's prescriber to build a medication schedule that accounts for school timing, and include medication administration in your teen's IHP (individualized health plan) so the school nurse can support it.

Eating Safely in a Teenager's World

The low-histamine diet is a common recommendation for MCAS, but applying it to a teenager's life requires flexibility and honesty about what is realistic. A perfectly restrictive diet that a teen refuses to follow is less effective than a moderately careful approach that they can sustain.

High-histamine foods to reduce include aged cheeses, fermented products (yogurt, sauerkraut, soy sauce), cured or smoked meats, canned fish, vinegar-based dressings, leftover cooked proteins (histamine levels rise as food sits), and certain fruits (strawberries, citrus, tomatoes).

For school lunches, fresh-cooked proteins (chicken, turkey), fresh vegetables, rice, and safe fruits can form a reliable base. Insulated lunch containers that keep food cold reduce histamine development. Snack options like rice crackers, seed butters, fresh fruit (safe varieties), and homemade muffins give teens choices that fit into school culture without drawing excessive attention.

Social eating is one of the hardest aspects of MCAS for teenagers. Birthday parties, restaurant outings, school events, and dating all revolve around food. Rather than avoiding these situations entirely, help your teen develop strategies: eating before events, bringing safe snacks, learning to scan menus for lower-risk options, and practicing brief, confident explanations ("I have a medical condition that means I react to certain foods. It is not a preference, it is a medical thing. Thanks for understanding.").

One caution: in teenagers, particularly girls, the intersection of dietary restriction and eating disorder risk demands attention. Restrictive eating for medical reasons can, in some teens, merge with or mask disordered eating patterns. If your teen's relationship with food shifts from cautious to fearful, rigid, or accompanied by shame, involve a nutritionist or therapist experienced in both MCAS and eating disorders.

Preparing for the Worst

All teens with MCAS who have experienced or are at risk for anaphylaxis should carry two auto-injectors of epinephrine at all times. The school nurse should have additional epinephrine available, and your teen's emergency care plan should specify when and how to administer it.

Train your teen to use the auto-injector themselves. Train their close friends. Train their teachers. Anaphylaxis does not wait for the school nurse to arrive.

Action Step: Create a MCAS flare kit for your teen to keep in their backpack: antihistamines (both H1 and H2), epinephrine auto-injector, a medical alert card listing diagnoses and emergency contacts, a bottle of water, and a safe snack. Review the kit monthly to replace expired medications.

In a Nutshell

MCAS management in adolescents requires a three-pronged approach: trigger identification and avoidance, layered medication protocols, and anaphylaxis preparedness.

Triggers are individual, inconsistent, and often invisible. School environments present specific challenges that should be addressed in accommodation plans.

Medication protocols should be timed around the school day. Sedating medications belong in the evening. Preventive medications require consistent timing that may need school nurse support.

Dietary management should be realistic and sustainable, not perfectly restrictive. Social eating strategies preserve your teen's social life while managing risk.

Every teen with MCAS who has had or is at risk for anaphylaxis must carry epinephrine and know how to use it. The people around them should know too.

Chapter 7 Make All Three Work Together

Sebastian's mother kept three binders in her car. One was labeled POTS, filled with cardiology notes, tilt table results, and medication logs. One was labeled EDS, with physical therapy records, geneticist letters, and a list of every joint that had ever subluxated. One was labeled MCAS, containing allergy workup results, flare photographs, and a food reaction diary.

Each binder was thorough. Each represented years of advocacy. But the three binders had never been in the same room at the same time during a medical appointment.

That was the problem. Sebastian's cardiologist managed his POTS without knowing that his fludrocortisone might be worsening his MCAS-driven fluid retention and swelling. His physical therapist pushed exercise to help his POTS without realizing that aerobic activity above a certain threshold triggered mast cell flares. His allergist adjusted his antihistamine doses without considering that the sedating effects were compounding the fatigue from his beta-blocker.

Each specialist was doing their job. But nobody was looking at the whole picture.

The trifecta is not three separate problems that happen to share a body. It is a single interconnected system in which every treatment decision affects all three conditions simultaneously. Managing it well requires coordination, communication, and a willingness to accept trade-offs.

When Treatments Work Against Each Other

The most common treatment conflict in the trifecta is the tension between POTS management and MCAS management.

POTS treatment calls for increased sodium and fluid intake to expand blood volume. This is foundational and effective. But some

MCAS patients find that high sodium worsens their symptoms, particularly bloating and GI distress, because mast cells in the gut are already activated and the additional sodium increases osmotic load on an inflamed system.

POTS treatment calls for regular aerobic exercise. Exercise is the strongest long-term intervention for POTS. But exercise is also a potent mast cell trigger. Many teens with the trifecta find that the very activities prescribed to improve their POTS cause MCAS flares: flushing, hives, GI distress, tachycardia from histamine release (not just from autonomic dysfunction), and in some cases, exercise-induced anaphylaxis.

EDS management calls for joint stabilization through physical therapy and strengthened muscles. But the deconditioning caused by POTS (because standing and moving feel terrible) and the exercise intolerance caused by MCAS create barriers to the consistent physical therapy that EDS requires.

The solution is not to choose one condition to treat and ignore the others. The solution is to find the protocol that moves all three conditions in the right direction simultaneously, even if progress is slow and compromises are necessary.

For the sodium-MCAS conflict, try electrolyte solutions that are lower in sodium per dose but taken more frequently, rather than large sodium boluses. Some teens tolerate sodium better when it comes from food rather than supplements, and when it is paired with adequate magnesium.

For the exercise-MCAS conflict, pretreat with antihistamines (both H1 and H2) 30 to 60 minutes before exercise. Start at very low intensity and increase gradually. Exercise in cool environments. Stop at the first sign of mast cell activation (flushing, itching, GI distress) and use rescue antihistamines if needed. Over time, as the cardiovascular system strengthens and mast cells are better controlled with baseline medications, exercise tolerance typically improves.

For the deconditioning-pain cycle, begin with recumbent exercises that place minimal stress on unstable joints and do not require standing.

Aquatic therapy (pool temperature must be warm enough to avoid cold triggers but cool enough to avoid heat triggers, typically 84 to 88 degrees Fahrenheit) can address POTS reconditioning, EDS stabilization, and MCAS trigger avoidance simultaneously.

The Quarterback Model

Every trifecta teen needs one provider who sees the whole picture. This does not mean one provider who manages all three conditions, that level of expertise is rare. It means one provider who receives copies of every specialist note, reviews the complete medication list for interactions and contradictions, and asks the question that specialists working in silos do not ask: "How is this treatment affecting the other two conditions?"

This coordinating provider is often the teen's primary care physician, though it can also be an adolescent medicine specialist, a nurse practitioner with interest in complex chronic illness, or, in some specialized centers, a physician who focuses specifically on the trifecta.

Regardless of who fills this role, the system works only if information flows. After every specialist appointment, send a summary to the coordinator. Before making any medication change, confirm that it has been reviewed in the context of all three conditions. If the coordinator does not know about a recommendation, they cannot flag potential conflicts.

Action Step: Identify your teen's care coordinator. If no single provider currently fills this role, ask your primary care physician if they are willing to serve as the central point of communication for all specialist recommendations. Provide them with a one-page medication list and a one-paragraph summary of current treatment goals for each condition.

When Everything Flares at Once

Multi-system flares are the most frightening part of the trifecta. Your teen wakes up with a racing heart, aching joints, hives across their torso, and nausea so severe they cannot eat. Is the POTS driving the nausea? Is the MCAS driving the tachycardia through histamine-mediated vasodilation? Is the EDS pain triggering a stress response that activates both POTS and MCAS?

The honest answer is usually "all of the above." In a trifecta flare, the conditions amplify each other. The challenge is deciding which condition to address first.

A practical triage approach starts with safety. If there are signs of anaphylaxis (throat tightness, difficulty breathing, severe drop in blood pressure), administer epinephrine and call emergency services. This takes priority over everything else.

If the flare is severe but not anaphylactic, address the condition causing the most acute danger or distress first. Severe tachycardia and presyncope call for immediate POTS interventions: lie down, elevate legs, hydrate with electrolytes, apply abdominal compression. Active mast cell symptoms (progressive hives, GI cramping, flushing) call for rescue antihistamines and mast cell stabilizers. Acute joint instability or subluxation calls for gentle repositioning, bracing, ice, and rest.

The trifecta flare toolkit should be accessible at home and in your teen's school bag. It should contain: antihistamines (H1 and H2), epinephrine auto-injector, electrolyte packets, water, a small blood pressure/heart rate monitor, cold packs, elastic bandage wraps for joint support, a medical information card, and emergency contact numbers.

When to Go to the Emergency Room

Emergency room visits for trifecta teens can be frustrating because most ER physicians are unfamiliar with these conditions. But certain situations require emergency evaluation regardless.

Go to the ER if your teen experiences anaphylaxis or suspected anaphylaxis (even after administering epinephrine), syncope with injury, heart rate sustained above 170 bpm that does not respond to lying down and fluids, severe dehydration with inability to keep fluids down, or a joint dislocation that you cannot reduce.

Bring a one-page medical summary that lists all three diagnoses, current medications, allergies, recent specialist contacts, and a brief description of the trifecta for the treating physician. Many parents of trifecta teens keep laminated copies of this document in their wallet, their teen's backpack, and the glove compartment.

Expect that the ER physician may not know what MCAS is. Be prepared to explain it calmly and clearly. Expect that they may want to attribute symptoms to anxiety. Bring your documentation. Remain polite but firm.

In a Nutshell

The trifecta is not three separate conditions. It is a single interconnected system in which every treatment decision affects all three conditions simultaneously.

Treatment conflicts are common. Salt loading for POTS may worsen MCAS gut symptoms. Exercise for POTS may trigger MCAS flares. Deconditioning from POTS and MCAS prevents the physical therapy that EDS requires.

Solutions involve creative compromise: pretreating with antihistamines before exercise, using aquatic therapy to address all three conditions simultaneously, and adjusting sodium delivery methods based on individual tolerance.

Every trifecta teen needs a care coordinator who sees the whole picture and reviews all treatment recommendations for cross-condition conflicts.

Multi-system flares require triage: address safety first, then the condition causing the most acute distress, then support the others. A prepared flare toolkit and a laminated medical summary can make emergencies less chaotic and ER visits more productive.

The goal is not perfection. The goal is a management system that moves all three conditions in the right direction, even slowly, even with setbacks. Progress in the trifecta is measured in weeks and months, not days. And it is real.

PART III CONQUERING SCHOOL WITH THE TRIFECTA

Chapter 8 Claim Your Legal Protections

Margot's mother walked into the 504 meeting with a folder of medical records, a letter from the pediatric cardiologist, and a printed list of accommodations she had found on a dysautonomia support website. She sat across from the school psychologist, the assistant principal, and Margot's guidance counselor. She expected a conversation. What she got was a wall.

The assistant principal spoke first. "Margot's grades are passing. She does not qualify for any special services."

Margot's mother tried to explain. Her daughter had missed 34 days of school in the past semester. She fainted in the hallway twice. She spent most lunch periods in the nurse's office because standing in the cafeteria line made her heart race above 140. She could not carry her backpack up the stairs without her knees buckling. She was surviving school, not succeeding in it.

"Passing grades mean she is accessing her education," the psychologist replied. "A 504 plan is not necessary."

This is one of the most common and most damaging misunderstandings in educational law as it applies to chronically ill students. Passing grades do not disqualify a student from a 504 plan. A student does not need to be failing to deserve protection. The legal standard is not academic failure. The legal standard is that a physical or mental impairment substantially limits one or more major life activities. For a teen with POTS, EDS, and MCAS, multiple major life activities are affected: standing, walking, breathing, eating, concentrating, learning, and caring for oneself (U.S. Department of Education, Office for Civil Rights, 2020).

Margot's mother did not know this at the time. She left the meeting feeling defeated, and Margot spent the rest of the year without any formal protections. It was not until summer, when she found an education advocate through a parent support group, that she learned the school had been wrong. Margot returned in the fall with a 504 plan that included 22 specific accommodations. Her attendance improved. Her grades went from passing to strong. And she stopped spending her lunch period lying on the nurse's cot.

The law is on your side. But the law only helps you if you know what it says and how to use it. This chapter will teach you the legal frameworks that protect your teen, how to activate them, and what to do when schools resist.

Section 504 Gives Broad Medical Protection

Section 504 of the Rehabilitation Act of 1973 is a federal civil rights law that prohibits discrimination against people with disabilities in any program receiving federal funding. Every public school in the United States receives federal funding. Every public school is therefore bound by Section 504.

To qualify for a 504 plan, a student must have a physical or mental impairment that substantially limits one or more major life activities. The 2008 amendments to the Americans with Disabilities Act broadened this definition significantly. Major life activities now include not only learning, reading, and concentrating, but also standing, walking, eating, sleeping, breathing, thinking, communicating, and the operation of major bodily functions, including neurological, cardiovascular, immune, and digestive functions (ADA Amendments Act, 2008).

Look at that list through the lens of the trifecta.

POTS substantially limits standing, walking, concentrating, thinking, and cardiovascular function. EDS substantially limits walking, lifting, bending, and musculoskeletal function. MCAS substantially limits eating, breathing, immune function, and digestive function.

Any one of these conditions can qualify a student for 504 protection. A teen with all three has an overwhelming case.

The school cannot consider the effects of medication or treatment when determining eligibility. If your teen's POTS is partially controlled by fludrocortisone and salt loading, the school must evaluate the impairment as it would present without those interventions. This is a point many schools get wrong, and it is worth stating clearly during the meeting.

The application process begins with a written request. You can submit a letter or email to the school's 504 coordinator (often the school psychologist or a designated administrator) requesting that your child be evaluated for a 504 plan. Include your teen's diagnoses, a brief description of how the conditions affect school participation, and a note that you are requesting this evaluation under Section 504 of the Rehabilitation Act. The school is required to respond.

Action Step: Write the request letter today. It does not need to be long. Three paragraphs will do: who your child is, what conditions they have, and that you are requesting a 504 evaluation. Date it. Send it by email so you have a digital record. The clock starts when the school receives your request.

When a 504 Plan Is Not Enough

A 504 plan provides accommodations. It adjusts the environment so your teen can access the same curriculum as their peers. But it does not change what your teen is taught or how they are taught. If your teen needs specialized instruction, modified curriculum, related services like occupational therapy or counseling, or a level of support that goes beyond accommodation, an Individualized Education Program (IEP) may be the stronger option.

IEP eligibility falls under the Individuals with Disabilities Education Act (IDEA). To qualify, a student must have a disability that falls under one of 13 categories recognized by IDEA and must need specially designed instruction as a result. For teens with the trifecta, the most relevant category is usually "Other Health Impairment" (OHI), which covers students whose chronic or acute health problems result in limited strength, alertness, or responsiveness that adversely affects educational performance (IDEA, 2004).

The word "adversely" is broader than "failing." A student whose concentration is impaired by brain fog, whose stamina is depleted by chronic pain, whose attendance is disrupted by unpredictable flares, and whose participation is limited by physical restrictions is experiencing adverse educational effects even if their report card shows passing marks.

To request an IEP evaluation, submit a written request to the school's special education department. The school must respond within a defined timeframe (typically 15 school days to decide on evaluation, then 60 calendar days to complete it, though state timelines vary). The evaluation should include input from your teen's medical providers, and you have the right to provide outside evaluations and medical documentation.

One important distinction: a 504 plan and an IEP are not mutually exclusive. Some students have both. A teen might have an IEP that addresses academic modifications and specialized instruction, and a 504 plan or individualized health plan that addresses medical accommodations and emergency protocols. The combination can provide the most thorough protection.

Consider what happened to Julian. His 504 plan covered extra time on tests and elevator access. But Julian's POTS was severe enough that he missed 40% of school days during flare periods. He needed homebound instruction during those periods, a modified curriculum that accounted for his fragmented attendance, and occupational therapy to address the fine motor difficulties caused by his EDS. A 504 plan could not provide those services. An IEP could and did.

Health Plans Protect Your Teen's Body at School

Even with a 504 plan or IEP in place, your teen needs two additional documents that address medical safety specifically: an Individualized Health Plan (IHP) and an Emergency Care Plan (ECP).

The IHP is developed by the school nurse in collaboration with the family and the teen's healthcare providers. It outlines the day-to-day medical management your teen needs during school hours: medication schedules, vital sign monitoring, dietary requirements, activity restrictions, and protocols for managing predictable symptoms like presyncope, joint instability, or GI distress.

The ECP addresses emergencies. For a teen with the trifecta, the relevant emergencies include syncope (fainting), joint dislocation or subluxation, and anaphylaxis or severe mast cell activation. Each emergency should have a clearly written protocol that any staff member can follow, including substitute teachers, cafeteria workers, and coaches who may not know your teen.

A strong ECP for a trifecta teen includes the following elements: the student's name, photo, grade, and classroom; diagnoses and a brief description of each condition; the names and contact information for parents, primary care physician, cardiologist, and allergist/immunologist; a step-by-step response protocol for each type of emergency; medication names, doses, and locations (nurse's office, backpack, classroom); and clear instructions for when to call 911 versus when to call the parent.

As we discussed in Chapter 6, every teen with MCAS who is at risk for anaphylaxis should have epinephrine accessible at school. The ECP should specify where the auto-injectors are stored, who is trained to administer them, and the sequence of actions after administration (call 911, call parent, position student, monitor breathing).

Action Step: Schedule a meeting with the school nurse before the school year begins (or as soon as possible if the year is underway). Bring your teen's medication list, a letter from each treating specialist describing the condition and school-relevant symptoms, and a draft of the emergency protocols you want in place. The nurse is your closest ally inside the building. Invest time in that relationship early.

Fight Back When Schools Say No

Schools deny 504 requests, minimize accommodations, fail to implement agreed-upon plans, and sometimes simply ignore the law. This is not always malicious. Often, it reflects a lack of training, limited resources, or genuine unfamiliarity with the trifecta conditions. But the effect on your teen is the same regardless of the reason.

Document everything. Every email, every meeting, every phone call. After a verbal conversation with a teacher or administrator, follow up with an email that summarizes what was discussed and what was agreed upon. "Thank you for meeting with me today. I want to confirm that we agreed Coralie will have elevator access starting Monday and that the PE teacher will be notified by Friday. Please let me know if I have captured this incorrectly." This creates a paper trail that protects you if the school later claims the conversation never happened.

If the school denies your 504 request, ask for the denial in writing with specific reasons. The school must evaluate your child. If they refuse to evaluate, you can file a complaint with the Office for Civil Rights (OCR) at the U.S. Department of Education. OCR complaints can be filed online and do not require an attorney.

If the school has a 504 plan but is not following it, document the failures. A plan that is not implemented is a plan that does not protect your child. Contact the 504 coordinator in writing, state which accommodations are not being provided, and request an immediate remedy. If the response is inadequate, an OCR complaint or a request for mediation through your school district may be your next step.

If the dispute involves an IEP, you have additional protections under IDEA, including the right to an independent educational evaluation, mediation, and a due process hearing. Due process hearings are formal and may benefit from legal representation.

When should you involve an education attorney? Consider it when the school has repeatedly failed to implement the plan, when the school refuses to evaluate your child despite clear medical documentation, when your teen's health or safety is at risk, or when the district's behavior suggests a pattern of denying services to students with medical disabilities. Many education attorneys offer free initial consultations, and some take cases on a contingent or reduced-fee basis.

A plan on paper is only as strong as the people who enforce it. You are that person.

Summary

Section 504 protects any student whose medical condition substantially limits a major life activity. Passing grades do not disqualify your teen. The school cannot consider the effects of treatment when evaluating eligibility.

An IEP under IDEA provides stronger protections when your teen needs specialized instruction, modified curriculum, or related services beyond what accommodations alone can offer. The category "Other Health Impairment" covers the trifecta.

An Individualized Health Plan and Emergency Care Plan address your teen's medical safety at school. They are separate from the 504/IEP and should be developed with the school nurse.

When schools deny, minimize, or fail to implement protections, documentation is your strongest tool. OCR complaints, mediation, due process hearings, and education attorneys are available when the school does not meet its legal obligations.

The law was written for students like yours. Use it.

Chapter 9 Get Accommodations That Work

Ines had a 504 plan. On paper, it looked thorough. Extended time on tests. Preferential seating. Permission to carry a water bottle. Excused absences for medical appointments.

On paper, it was fine. In practice, it was useless.

The extended time was granted, but the testing room was on the third floor with no elevator and no air conditioning. Ines arrived to every test with her heart pounding from the stairs and her head swimming from the heat. The preferential seating placed her in the front row, where standing up to leave for the bathroom meant walking past every classmate while they watched. The water bottle was allowed, but the electrolyte powder she needed to mix into it was confiscated because it was classified as "outside food." And the excused absences protected her grade but did nothing to help her learn the material she missed during flares.

Ines's plan was not designed by someone who understood her conditions. It was assembled from a generic template and applied without attention to the specific ways POTS, EDS, and MCAS affect a teenager's school day. The accommodations looked reasonable on a form. They failed in a hallway, a classroom, and a stairwell.

The difference between a 504 plan that works and one that does not is specificity. General accommodations help generally. Condition-specific accommodations, designed around the actual mechanics of your teen's symptoms, can change the entire school experience. This chapter breaks down the accommodations that make the most difference for trifecta teens, organized by the area of school life they affect.

Attendance That Reflects Medical Reality

Chronic illness does not follow a school calendar. Flares are unpredictable. Bad days cluster. Mornings are often the worst time for

POTS. And the standard school response to excessive absences, referral to truancy services, threat of grade penalties, or mandatory parent conferences framed as disciplinary meetings, can turn a medical problem into a legal one.

Your teen's plan should include a modified attendance policy that distinguishes between medically documented absences and unexcused absences. The plan should state that absences related to the documented medical conditions will not count toward truancy thresholds or trigger automatic disciplinary referrals.

But attendance protection alone does not solve the problem. If your teen misses 30% of school, they are missing 30% of instruction. The plan must also address how missed content will be delivered.

Homebound instruction, sometimes called home hospital teaching, provides a certified teacher who comes to the home during extended absences. This service is typically available when a physician certifies that the student cannot attend school for a defined period (often three weeks or more). It is a safety net, not a replacement for in-person school. The hours are limited (often five to ten hours per week), and the instruction may cover only core subjects.

For teens whose attendance is inconsistent rather than completely absent, a flexible scheduling arrangement may be more effective. Late start times can accommodate the morning severity of POTS symptoms. Half-day schedules allow the teen to attend during their best hours and complete remaining work at home. Reduced course loads, taking four courses instead of six, prevent overwhelm during semesters when health is unstable.

Oscar's family negotiated a hybrid schedule: three days in school and two days working from home through the school's virtual learning platform. This arrangement let Oscar attend his most demanding classes in person while completing independent work at home on days when his symptoms were poorly controlled. His attendance record improved because he was present more consistently on the days he attended, rather than leaving early three times a week.

Action Step: Before your next 504 meeting, calculate your teen's actual attendance over the past semester. Note which class periods are most affected (mornings are usually hardest for POTS). Propose a specific schedule modification with days, times, and a plan for making up missed content. Specific proposals get better responses than general requests for "flexibility."

Design the Physical Environment for Safety

The physical layout of a school building creates daily obstacles for trifecta teens that healthy students never notice. Stairs raise heart rates and threaten unstable joints. Long hallways require sustained walking and standing. Classrooms vary in temperature, air quality, and seating. Lockers may be in the wrong location, too high, or too far from classrooms.

Elevator access should be automatic for any student with POTS or EDS. A key or code should be issued to the student and included in their 504 plan. The plan should also note that the student may be accompanied by a friend (isolation in elevators increases the stigma that makes many teens refuse to use them, as we saw with Clara's backpack story in Chapter 1).

Classroom seating should be near the door so the student can leave quietly for the bathroom, the nurse's office, or simply to stand in the hallway for a moment when symptoms spike. An ergonomic chair or the ability to alternate between sitting and standing helps teens with EDS who develop pain from sustained sitting in standard desks. Some students benefit from a footrest or a compression cushion.

Temperature control matters more than most schools realize. Heat is a common trigger for both POTS and MCAS flares. If the classroom is poorly ventilated or runs warm, the student should be relocated to a cooler room or a portable fan should be provided. Fragrance-free policies in the student's immediate area can reduce MCAS triggers from perfumes, body sprays, scented hand sanitizers, and cleaning products, which are ubiquitous in school hallways.

Locker placement should be near the student's primary classrooms and at a comfortable height. Duplicate textbook sets (one at home, one in the classroom) eliminate the need to carry heavy books. A rolling backpack or permission to use a cart removes the joint stress of a loaded bag.

Bathroom access requires a permanent hall pass or an arrangement with each teacher that allows the student to leave without asking. For teens with MCAS who experience sudden GI distress, or teens with POTS who need to use the bathroom frequently due to high fluid intake, the delay of raising a hand and waiting for permission can be the difference between dignity and humiliation.

Protect Academic Performance During Flares

Brain fog from POTS is not a metaphor. It is reduced cerebral blood flow causing measurable impairment in attention, processing speed, working memory, and word retrieval. It worsens with dehydration, poor sleep, warm rooms, and prolonged standing. It can fluctuate within a single class period.

Extended time on tests and assignments is the most commonly granted academic accommodation, and it is usually insufficient by itself. The testing environment matters as much as the time. Tests should be administered in a quiet, cool room where the student can have water, electrolyte drinks, and salty snacks. The student should be allowed to stand, walk, or change position during the test. If brain fog is severe on a testing day, the plan should allow the test to be rescheduled.

Note-taking accommodations address the reality that many trifecta teens cannot both listen and write simultaneously, especially when brain fog is present or when EDS makes handwriting painful. Options include peer note-takers, teacher-provided notes or outlines, permission to record lectures on a phone or laptop, and use of a laptop for all written work.

Modified assignment deadlines during flares prevent the devastating cycle of falling behind, feeling overwhelmed, and then missing more school due to the stress of an unmanageable workload. The plan should specify that during documented flare periods, assignment deadlines will be extended by a defined number of days (rather than leaving it to individual teacher discretion, which creates inconsistency).

Elio's 504 plan included a provision his mother fought hard to include: if Elio missed three or more consecutive days due to a medical flare, his teachers would collectively prioritize assignments, identifying which were most critical for learning and which could be reduced or excused. This prevented the pile-up that had previously buried him after every absence.

Redesign PE for the Trifecta Body

Physical education is the single most dangerous class period for many trifecta teens, and it is also the class where accommodations are most frequently resisted.

Standard PE activities, running, dodgeball, rope climbing, contact sports, circuit training in hot gymnasiums, can provoke syncope in POTS, dislocations in EDS, and anaphylaxis-like reactions in MCAS. A blanket PE waiver might seem like the safest option, but it carries its own cost. Exercise is the most effective long-term treatment for POTS, as we discussed in Chapter 4. Removing all physical activity from a trifecta teen's schedule can worsen deconditioning and delay recovery.

The better approach is a modified PE program built around what the teen can do safely. Recumbent cycling, swimming in a temperature-controlled pool, gentle yoga with joint protection modifications, walking at the teen's own pace, and upper-body strength training with light weights can all satisfy PE requirements while supporting the teen's health rather than undermining it.

The 504 plan should specify the type of exercise, the intensity limits, the environmental conditions (cool gymnasium, access to water, proximity to the nurse's office), and the criteria for stopping activity (heart rate exceeding a specified threshold, onset of flushing or hives, joint pain above a defined level). It should also specify who monitors the activity. A PE teacher who does not understand POTS may interpret a teen sitting on the gym floor as laziness rather than presyncope.

Alternative PE credit, including documented home exercise logs, sessions with a physical therapist, or participation in community adaptive programs, should be available for periods when in-school PE is not feasible.

Action Step: Request a meeting with the PE teacher before the school year starts. Bring the physician's exercise prescription from Chapter 4. Walk through what your teen can and cannot do. Frame it as a partnership: you want your teen to be active, and you need the PE teacher's help making that safe.

Give Your Teen Access to Food and Fluids

It sounds simple. A water bottle on the desk. A snack in the backpack. But in many schools, these basic tools of trifecta management are treated as violations of classroom rules.

Water and electrolyte drinks should be allowed in every classroom, every period, without exception. POTS management requires continuous hydration, not a sip at the water fountain between classes. The 504 plan should state that the student may have a water bottle on their desk at all times and may refill it without restriction.

Salty snacks serve a medical purpose for teens with POTS: they support blood volume expansion and prevent the sodium depletion that worsens orthostatic symptoms. The plan should allow the student to eat small snacks during class, kept in a desk drawer or backpack, consumed quietly and without disruption.

Cafeteria accommodations for teens with MCAS may include permission to bring home-prepared meals, access to ingredient information for school-prepared food, a designated allergen-aware eating space, and communication of specific food sensitivities to cafeteria staff. Some families find it most practical to have the teen eat a packed lunch in the nurse's office or a quiet classroom rather than attempting to manage the sensory and chemical exposure of a crowded cafeteria.

Medication administration during the school day must be addressed in the IHP and the 504 plan. Specify which medications the teen takes during school hours, the timing, the location (nurse's office or self-carry), and the procedures for documentation. Many states allow students to self-carry and self-administer certain medications (including epinephrine and asthma inhalers) with physician authorization and parental consent.

Valeria's school initially refused to let her carry her antihistamines in her backpack, insisting that all medications be stored in the nurse's office. But the nurse's office was in a separate building, and during a mast cell flare in the science lab, the ten-minute walk to retrieve her medication turned a manageable reaction into one that required an ambulance. After that incident, the plan was revised to allow Valeria to carry a rescue kit in her backpack at all times.

Summary

Accommodations only work when they are designed around the specific mechanics of your teen's conditions, not assembled from a generic list.

Attendance accommodations should include modified absence policies, homebound instruction protocols for extended flares, and flexible scheduling options that match your teen's best hours.

Physical environment modifications (elevator access, classroom seating, temperature control, bathroom passes, fragrance reduction) remove the daily obstacles that drain your teen's energy before learning can begin.

Academic protections (extended time in cool rooms, note-taking supports, flare-period deadline extensions, prioritized makeup work) address brain fog and unpredictable absences directly.

PE should be modified, not eliminated. A physician-prescribed exercise plan replaces standard PE with activities that support recovery instead of causing harm.

Food and fluid access, including water bottles, electrolyte drinks, salty snacks, safe meal options, and medication self-carry, must be explicitly written into the plan to prevent staff from treating medical needs as rule violations.

The best accommodation plan is the one your teen's teachers actually understand and follow. Share it with every staff member who interacts with your child, and check in monthly to confirm it is working.

Chapter 10 Partner with the School Nurse

Gabriel's school nurse, Mrs. Chen, had been a registered nurse for 22 years. She had managed students with diabetes, epilepsy, severe food allergies, and asthma. She had handled emergency situations calmly and saved at least two young lives with her quick response to anaphylactic reactions. She was, by any measure, an excellent school nurse.

She had never heard of POTS. She had a vague understanding of Ehlers-Danlos syndrome from a nursing textbook chapter on rare genetic conditions. She had never encountered the term "mast cell activation syndrome" outside of a continuing education module she had skimmed three years earlier.

When Gabriel's mother arrived in September with three pages of medical documentation and a request for daily blood pressure monitoring, Mrs. Chen looked at the paperwork and said, honestly, "I am going to need some help understanding this."

That honesty was the best possible starting point.

Most school nurses have strong clinical foundations but limited exposure to the trifecta conditions. A 2023 survey by the National Association of School Nurses found that fewer than 15% of school nurses reported receiving any training on dysautonomia during their educational preparation (NASN, 2023). MCAS is not covered in most nursing school curricula. EDS appears briefly in genetics or musculoskeletal units and is rarely connected to its systemic effects.

This is not a criticism of school nurses. It is a description of the training gap that families must bridge. The school nurse is the single most important in-building advocate your teen can have. But they can only advocate effectively if they understand the conditions. This chapter is about building that partnership.

Teach Before You Ask

The instinct when your teen starts a new school year is to arrive with a list of demands: daily blood pressure readings, medication at 11:15, emergency epinephrine, cool room access, restricted PE. The demands are all reasonable. But leading with demands before the nurse understands the "why" behind them creates resistance rather than partnership.

Start by educating. Before the school year begins or as soon after diagnosis as possible, request a meeting with the school nurse. Do not bring your accommodation list first. Bring information.

Prepare a one-page summary for each condition that covers: the name and a plain-language explanation, how it affects your specific teen (not the condition in general, but your child's presentation), the symptoms the nurse is most likely to see during the school day, what the nurse should do when those symptoms appear, and what constitutes an emergency. Keep each summary to a single page. Nurses are busy. They manage hundreds of students. Concise, clear information is far more likely to be read, remembered, and taped to the wall behind their desk.

Offer to share links to short educational videos or one-page clinical summaries from Dysautonomia International, the Ehlers-Danlos Society, and the Mast Cell Disease Society. These organizations produce nurse-friendly materials that take minutes to review and carry clinical credibility.

Then, once the nurse understands the conditions, present your accommodation requests in the context of that understanding. "Now that you know Gabriel's heart rate can spike above 140 just from standing in the hallway, you can see why he needs the option to lie down in your office during the school day" is a far stronger request than "Gabriel needs rest breaks."

Build Condition-Specific Protocols

Once the nurse understands the trifecta, work together to develop written protocols that the nurse (and any substitute nurse or front-office staff) can follow during the school day.

A POTS monitoring protocol should specify how often the nurse checks the student's vitals (heart rate and blood pressure), what the target ranges are, what symptoms indicate the student should rest, and what symptoms indicate the student should be sent home or to the emergency room. For many trifecta teens, a daily morning check-in with the nurse to assess baseline status is helpful. If the teen arrives already tachycardic and symptomatic, the nurse can notify teachers early and prepare for a likely shortened day.

An EDS first response protocol should cover the most common orthopedic events the nurse is likely to encounter: finger and hand subluxations (the student can often guide the nurse through self-reduction), knee and ankle instability (bracing, ice, rest), shoulder subluxation or dislocation (sling, ice, parent notification, and medical evaluation if the student cannot reduce it), and general joint pain management (ice, positioning, pain medication if authorized). The protocol should also note that standard first aid advice ("walk it off" or "stretch it out") can worsen EDS injuries.

An MCAS emergency protocol should mirror the anaphylaxis protocols the nurse already knows, with the additional understanding that mast cell activation episodes can present differently from typical allergic reactions. The protocol should include the location of the student's epinephrine, the criteria for administration (any two or more of the following: progressive hives, flushing with GI distress, throat tightness, dizziness with blood pressure drop, difficulty breathing), the post-administration steps (call 911, position the student, notify parents, prepare for a second dose), and a clear statement that antihistamines alone may not be sufficient during a severe episode.

Medication storage and administration procedures should specify which medications are stored in the nurse's office, which the student self-carries (as discussed in Chapter 9 with Valeria's story), the timing and dosing of each, and documentation requirements. Many school districts require physician authorization forms for every medication administered at school, so complete these forms before the school year begins to avoid delays.

Action Step: After your meeting with the school nurse, write a brief email summarizing what was discussed and what protocols will be developed. Attach the one-page condition summaries. Ask the nurse to share them with the front office staff and any health aides who cover during the nurse's absence. Documentation protects both your teen and the nurse.

Extend Protocols Beyond the Nurse's Office

The school nurse is the center of the medical safety network, but your teen spends most of the day outside the nurse's office. Protocols only protect your teen if the people around them know the protocols.

Field trips are a common blind spot. When Paloma's eighth-grade class went to a science museum, the chaperone was a parent volunteer who knew nothing about POTS, EDS, or MCAS. The building was warm, the walking was continuous, and there was no plan for what to do if Paloma became symptomatic. She fainted in the geology exhibit. The chaperone called 911 instead of following the school's own emergency protocol, which would have directed her to lay Paloma down, elevate her legs, and offer fluids. The ambulance ride was unnecessary and cost the family $1,200.

Work with the nurse to create a field trip protocol that travels with your teen. It should be a laminated card, small enough to fit in a chaperone's pocket, listing the student's conditions, the key "do this first" steps for each type of event, emergency contacts, and the location of medications in the student's bag. Every adult supervising the trip should receive a copy.

Coaches and extracurricular supervisors are another gap. If your teen participates in any after-school activity, the supervising adult needs a brief version of the medical plan. Theater directors, band instructors, club advisors, and coaches may all encounter situations where your teen's conditions present symptoms. A drama rehearsal in a hot auditorium, a marching band practice in the sun, or an art room filled with solvent fumes can all provoke a trifecta response.

The nurse can serve as the bridge to these staff members, but the initial information often needs to come from the family. Prepare a half-page summary (simpler than the one you give the nurse) that any non-medical adult can read in two minutes and act on. It should answer three questions: What might happen? What should I do first? Who should I call?

Ines's mother created a wallet-sized card for every adult in her daughter's life at school, from the cafeteria monitor to the debate team coach. It read: "Ines has three medical conditions that can cause fainting, allergic-type reactions, and joint injuries. If she tells you she feels unwell, believe her. Let her sit or lie down immediately. Give her water. Call the nurse or call me. Do not tell her to push through it." Simple. Clear. Life-changing for Ines, who had previously been told by a substitute teacher to "walk it off" during a presyncope episode.

Create Reliable Communication Systems

The best protocols in the world fail if the teen cannot reach the nurse when they need to, or if the nurse cannot communicate with teachers and parents when something changes.

Work with the nurse to establish a discrete signaling system your teen can use to indicate a problem during class. Options include a colored card placed on the desk, a brief text message to the nurse's office phone, or a standing pass arrangement where the student simply stands and walks to the nurse's office without needing to ask permission or explain the reason aloud. The key is discretion. Most teenagers would rather endure a symptom in silence than announce their medical need in front of 28 classmates.

Marcel's nurse developed a three-color card system with him. A green card placed on his desk meant "I am managing fine, no help needed." A yellow card meant "I need to come to the nurse's office within the next 15 minutes." A red card meant "I need to leave right now." Marcel's teachers all knew the system, and it allowed him to communicate his status without saying a word.

Substitute teacher notification is a gap that catches many families off guard. When the regular teacher is absent, the substitute often knows nothing about your teen's accommodations. The school should maintain a confidential list of students with medical plans, accessible to substitute teachers, that includes the student's name, condition summary, key accommodations, and emergency instructions. If the school does not have such a system, request that one be created and that your teen's information be included.

Parent-nurse communication should happen at a predictable rhythm. Some families check in weekly by email. Others find that a monthly brief exchange is sufficient. The nurse should contact you immediately if your teen experiences a medical event at school, is sent home early, or needs to use emergency medication. You should contact the nurse promptly if your teen's condition changes, if medication doses are adjusted, or if a flare period is anticipated.

The beginning of each semester is a natural time to update the partnership. Medications change over summer. New symptoms may have appeared. Growth spurts may have shifted your teen's EDS presentation. A five-minute email update before the first day of school gives the nurse current information without requiring a full meeting.

When the nurse-family partnership works well, it produces something that no accommodation plan can provide on its own: a trusted adult inside the building who knows your teen's body, notices changes, and can intervene before a bad hour becomes a bad day. Gabriel's nurse, Mrs. Chen, eventually became so attuned to his patterns that she could tell from his posture in the morning whether he would make it to fifth period or need to go home by lunch. That level of awareness came from months of honest communication, shared learning, and mutual respect.

Summary

The school nurse is your most powerful in-building ally, but they can only help if they understand your teen's conditions. Most school nurses have received minimal training on POTS, EDS, and MCAS.

Educate before you request. One-page condition summaries, brief videos from condition-specific organizations, and a personal meeting to discuss your teen's specific presentation build the foundation for effective collaboration.

Written protocols for POTS monitoring, EDS first response, and MCAS emergencies give the nurse (and any substitute) a clear guide for daily management and crisis response.

Discrete communication systems allow your teen to signal the nurse without announcing their condition to the classroom. Substitute teacher notification plans close a dangerous gap. Regular parent-nurse check-ins keep the partnership current.

Invest in the relationship with the school nurse. It is one of the highest-return investments you can make in your teen's school year.

Chapter 11 Succeed on Tests and Get Into College

Coralie took the SAT with no accommodations. She had not known she could request them. Her mother had not known either. So Coralie sat in a crowded auditorium with 200 other students on a warm Saturday morning, drinking from a small water bottle she had smuggled in her jacket pocket, fighting dizziness every time she looked up from the test booklet, and watching the clock with the sick awareness that her brain fog was getting worse by the hour.

She scored 150 points below her practice test average. When she got the results, she cried. Not because of the number, but because she knew the number did not represent what she could do. It represented what POTS, EDS, and MCAS had stolen from a four-hour testing window.

Coralie retook the SAT six months later with full accommodations: extended time (50% additional), extra breaks every 30 minutes, a small testing room with air conditioning, permission to bring water and electrolyte drinks, permission to bring snacks, and the option to stand or walk during breaks. Her score increased by 180 points.

The test did not change. The conditions did not change. What changed was that the testing environment stopped fighting her body. This is the purpose of accommodations, not to give an advantage, but to remove a disadvantage that has nothing to do with knowledge or ability.

Get the Testing Accommodations You Deserve

Both the College Board (which administers the SAT and AP exams) and ACT, Inc. have formal processes for requesting accommodations for students with disabilities. The process requires documentation, planning, and time. Start early.

For the College Board, accommodations requests are submitted through the student's school via the Services for Students with

Disabilities (SSD) online system. The school's SSD coordinator (usually the guidance counselor or 504 coordinator) initiates the request. Documentation must include a clinical diagnosis, a description of how the disability affects testing, a history of accommodations received at school (this is why your 504 plan matters, as it establishes a documented record of need), and, in some cases, a recent evaluation or physician letter.

For ACT, Inc., the process is similar. Requests are submitted through the student's school with supporting documentation from the school and healthcare providers.

The strongest applications connect three elements clearly: the medical diagnosis (POTS, EDS, MCAS), the functional limitation in a testing context (brain fog, fatigue, pain from prolonged sitting, risk of syncope, need for hydration and food, need for temperature control), and the specific accommodation that addresses that limitation (extended time, breaks, separate room, food and drink, ability to stand).

Begin the request process at least seven months before the intended test date. Late requests are reviewed but may not be approved in time. If your teen already has a 504 plan, the school's SSD coordinator can use the plan as supporting evidence. If the initial request is denied, you can appeal, and many families succeed on appeal with additional documentation from physicians.

AP exams follow the same College Board accommodation system as the SAT. If your teen is taking Advanced Placement classes, apply for AP accommodations at the same time as SAT accommodations. The approval typically covers both. AP exams are longer than the SAT (some last three hours or more), making extended time and break accommodations even more critical. Felix's family learned this the hard way when he had SAT accommodations approved but forgot to apply them to his AP exams. He took the AP Biology exam without breaks or extra time and scored a 2. He retook it the following year with full accommodations and earned a 4.

One option that many families overlook is test-optional admissions. A growing number of colleges no longer require SAT or ACT scores. For a teen whose trifecta symptoms make standardized testing especially difficult, even with accommodations, a test-optional school may reduce stress and allow the application to rest on transcript strength, essays, and extracurricular involvement instead. Research your teen's target schools early to determine their testing policies.

Action Step: Contact your teen's guidance counselor this week to ask about the SSD accommodation request timeline. If your teen does not yet have a 504 plan, as discussed in Chapter 8, establishing one now creates the documented history of need that testing organizations require.

Tell the Right Story in College Applications

College applications ask for transcripts, test scores, and personal essays. For a teen with the trifecta, the transcript may show grade dips, reduced course loads, incomplete semesters, or a shift from honors to standard-level classes. Without context, these records look like disengagement. With context, they look like resilience.

Most college applications include an "additional information" section where applicants can explain extenuating circumstances. This section is where your teen should briefly, clearly, and without melodrama, explain their medical conditions and how those conditions affected their academic record.

The explanation should be factual, forward-looking, and specific. "I was diagnosed with three chronic medical conditions in ninth grade that caused me to miss approximately 40% of school days during my sophomore year. I worked with my school to develop accommodations that allowed me to return to full attendance by junior year. My grades reflect the impact of this period, and my upward trend reflects my commitment to my education despite ongoing health management."

What the explanation should not be: a plea for pity, a detailed medical history, or a narrative that defines the applicant by their illness. Admissions officers want to see that the student has perspective on their circumstances and evidence of growth.

Letters of recommendation can also provide context. Ask a teacher who witnessed your teen's struggle and recovery to write about their persistence, their problem-solving, and their engagement with learning even during difficult periods. The teacher does not need to describe the medical conditions in detail. They need to describe the student.

Hugo's guidance counselor wrote a supplemental letter to three universities explaining, with the family's permission, that Hugo had spent his freshman year managing undiagnosed POTS that caused severe fatigue and frequent absences. The letter noted that once diagnosed and treated, Hugo's junior-year GPA was 3.7, up from 2.1 during the worst of his illness. All three universities offered admission.

Choose a College That Can Support You

Choosing a college with the trifecta involves all the usual considerations (academics, location, culture, cost) plus a layer of medical and logistical evaluation that healthy students never need to think about.

Campus accessibility is not just about wheelchair ramps. For a teen with POTS, it means evaluating how much walking is required between classes, the availability of elevators in classroom buildings, and the distance from dorms to dining halls and academic buildings. For a teen with EDS, it means understanding the terrain (hills, uneven sidewalks, ice in winter) and the physical demands of daily campus life. For a teen with MCAS, it means evaluating air quality, cleaning chemicals used in dorms, and whether the campus can accommodate fragrance-reduction requests.

Proximity to specialists matters. If your teen's current medical team is 400 miles from campus, find out what specialists are available near the university. Some families choose colleges within driving distance of the teen's established providers. Others identify new providers near the campus before the first semester and schedule transition appointments during summer orientation.

Disability services offices vary enormously in quality and responsiveness. During campus visits, schedule a meeting with disability services. Ask specific questions: How many students do you currently support with chronic medical conditions? What is the process for arranging absences during flares? Can accommodations be adjusted mid-semester if my health changes? What happens if a professor does not follow my accommodation plan?

Dorm accommodations for trifecta students may include a single room (reduced exposure to fragrances, allergens, and disrupted sleep), air conditioning (temperature control for POTS and MCAS), a medical-grade refrigerator (for medications and safe food storage), and placement on a lower floor near an elevator.

Meal plan accommodations should allow the student to work with dining services to identify safe food options or to opt out of the standard meal plan in favor of a kitchen-equipped living space where they can prepare their own food. Most colleges will work with students on this, but it requires early communication and medical documentation.

Martin visited six colleges before choosing one. He ranked them not by prestige or party scene, but by three criteria: distance from an established POTS cardiologist (under 90 minutes), quality of disability services (responsive emails, specific chronic illness experience, willingness to customize), and the availability of air-conditioned single dorm rooms on a ground floor. The college he chose was not his top academic pick. It was his top survival pick. He graduated in four years.

Know When to Take a Different Path

Not every teen with the trifecta will follow the traditional high school to four-year university timeline. And that is not a failure. It is a strategy.

A gap year between high school and college can serve a medical purpose. If your teen's conditions are unstable during senior year, starting college in crisis increases the risk of medical withdrawal, lost tuition, and the emotional blow of a failed attempt. A gap year focused on stabilizing health, establishing an exercise protocol, optimizing medications, and building self-management skills can make the difference between struggling through freshman year and succeeding in it.

Some teens benefit from starting at a community college while living at home. This allows them to test their ability to manage a course load independently while retaining the medical support system of home, access to established providers, and the safety net of family. Credits transfer to four-year institutions, and the financial cost of discovering that a full course load is too much is far lower at a community college than at a university.

Online degree programs have matured significantly in recent years and offer a legitimate path for students whose health makes consistent in-person attendance difficult. Accredited online programs allow students to attend class from bed on bad days, adjust their schedule around symptoms, and complete coursework during their best hours rather than conforming to a fixed campus schedule.

Zoe had planned to attend a university three states away. During her senior spring, her MCAS flared so severely that she was homebound for six weeks. Her family made the difficult decision to defer enrollment for a year. Zoe spent the gap year working with her medical team to identify her primary triggers, adjust her medication protocol, and build a consistent exercise routine. When she started college the following fall, she was more stable, more confident, and more prepared to manage independently than she would have been a year earlier.

The college timeline is not a race. The finish line is the same whether your teen crosses it at 22 or 25.

Action Step: If your teen is uncertain about the traditional college timeline, sit down together and list the medical, practical, and emotional factors that would make college more likely to succeed versus more likely to fail. Use the list to guide a conversation with the guidance counselor about whether gap years, community college, or online options deserve consideration.

Summary

Standardized testing accommodations are available for students with POTS, EDS, and MCAS. Extended time, breaks, separate rooms, food and drink access, and temperature control can dramatically improve scores. Start the request process at least seven months before the test date, and use the 504 plan as supporting evidence.

College applications should address the impact of chronic illness in the additional information section with brief, factual, forward-looking language. Teacher and counselor recommendation letters can provide context without defining the student by their diagnosis.

College selection for trifecta students requires evaluating campus accessibility, proximity to medical specialists, disability services quality, dorm accommodations (single room, air conditioning, medical refrigerator), and meal plan flexibility.

The right college is not always the most prestigious one. It is the one where your teen can manage their health, access their education, and build the life they want. Choose accordingly.

PART IV THE TEEN EXPERIENCE

Chapter 12 Your Body Is Telling the Truth

Elio sat in his pediatrician's office for the sixth time in four months. He was fifteen. He had missed 22 days of school. He was so tired that getting dressed in the morning felt like running a mile. His heart slammed against his ribs every time he stood up from his chair. His stomach rejected foods he had eaten his entire life. His skin broke out in red welts after gym class, and nobody could tell him why.

The pediatrician looked at the lab results, looked at Elio, and said, "Everything looks normal. Have you been feeling anxious about school?"

Elio stared at the floor. He was not anxious about school. He was anxious because his body was doing things he could not explain, and every adult he turned to told him nothing was wrong. He had started to wonder if maybe they were right. Maybe he was making it up. Maybe he was just weak. Maybe everyone felt this way and he was the only one who could not handle it.

He was wrong about all of that. But it took another eight months, two more doctors, and a mother who refused to stop asking questions before anyone told him so.

This chapter is for you. Not for your parents, not for your doctors, not for your teachers. For you, the teenager reading this in bed, or in a waiting room, or in the back seat of a car on the way to yet another appointment. If you have been told that your symptoms are stress, anxiety, growing pains, attention seeking, or all in your head, this chapter is going to tell you something different.

Your body is telling the truth. The dizziness is real. The fatigue is real. The pain is real. The brain fog, the racing heart, the flushing, the nausea, the joints that slip and pop and ache: all real. These are not personality flaws. They are medical conditions with names, with research behind them, and with treatments that can help.

You are not crazy. You are not lazy. And you are definitely not making it up.

Your Symptoms Have a Biological Explanation

Let us talk about why you feel terrible, in plain language, no medical jargon.

When you stand up and the room goes gray, that is not weakness. Your autonomic nervous system, the part of your brain that controls heart rate and blood pressure without you thinking about it, is not adjusting properly. Blood pools in your legs and gut instead of flowing up to your brain. Your heart speeds up trying to compensate. Your brain gets less oxygen than it needs. The result: dizziness, tunnel vision, brain fog, and sometimes fainting. That is POTS. It is a measurable, testable, diagnosable condition.

When your joints hurt for no obvious reason, when your fingers bend backward further than your friends' fingers, when your shoulder slides out of place while you are reaching for something on a shelf, that is not clumsiness. The connective tissue that holds your joints together is stretchier than it should be. It does not support your joints the way it is supposed to. That is EDS. It is genetic, it is structural, and it is not something you caused.

When your skin flushes and welts appear after you exercise, or when you walk into a room with strong perfume and your throat tightens and your stomach cramps, that is not an overreaction. Your mast cells, a type of immune cell, are releasing chemicals when they should not. They are treating harmless things like threats. That is MCAS. It is a real immune system malfunction, and it can be measured through lab tests taken at the right time.

Here is the part that confuses people, including doctors. Your symptoms are inconsistent. You might feel fine sitting down and terrible standing up. You might have a good day on Tuesday and be bedridden on Wednesday. You might look completely healthy in the morning and be unable to function by noon. This inconsistency is not evidence that you are faking. It is a hallmark of these conditions. POTS symptoms change with posture, hydration, temperature, and time of day. MCAS symptoms change with exposures that are often invisible. EDS pain changes with activity, weather, sleep quality, and hormonal cycles.

The inconsistency is the disease. It is not proof against it.

Action Step: The next time someone (a teacher, a friend, a relative, anyone) suggests your symptoms are not real, try this sentence: "I have three diagnosed medical conditions that cause my symptoms to fluctuate. It looks inconsistent from the outside, but my doctors have confirmed the diagnoses." You do not owe anyone a longer explanation than that.

Choose Who Gets Your Story

You do not have to tell everyone everything. Your medical conditions are your information to share on your terms, with the people you choose, in the amount of detail that feels right.

Some friends will get the full explanation. These are the people who have earned your trust, who listen without interrupting, and who do not try to fix you with advice they found on social media. Give them as much detail as you want. Let them ask questions. They may become your strongest allies.

Some friends will get the short version. "I have a chronic health condition that makes me tired and dizzy sometimes. I might need to sit down or leave early. It is not contagious and it is not a big deal, I just manage it." That is enough. If they push for more and you are not ready, it is fine to say, "I would rather not get into the details right now."

Some people will not get any explanation at all. The kid in your math class who made a joke about you leaving early does not deserve your medical history. The substitute teacher who raised an eyebrow when you used your elevator key does not need a diagnosis. You get to decide.

Handling disbelief is harder. When someone says "but you look fine" or "you were fine yesterday," the sting is real. It can make you question yourself, even when you know better. Here is what helps: stop trying to convince people who do not want to be convinced. You will waste energy you do not have. Instead, invest that energy in the people who believe you without proof.

Eloise found her people in an online support group for teens with POTS. "The first time I posted about brain fog during a test and fifteen people said 'same,' I actually cried," she said. "I had never talked to anyone my age who understood what it felt like." Online communities for teens with POTS, EDS, and MCAS can provide something that no amount of parental support can replace: the knowledge that someone your age, living your kind of life, understands exactly what you are going through.

Look for communities on platforms where you already spend time. Many are on Discord, Reddit, Instagram, and through organizations like Dysautonomia International and the Ehlers-Danlos Society. Some have teen-specific channels with age-appropriate moderation. Start by reading and observing before you post. Find the groups where the tone is supportive rather than competitive about suffering.

Protect Yourself Online

Online chronic illness communities can be a lifeline. They can also be a trap.

The helpful version looks like this: you find a group of teens who share practical tips, encourage each other on hard days, celebrate small wins, and treat their conditions as something they manage rather than something that defines them. You log off feeling less isolated and more informed.

The harmful version looks like this: you find a group where the culture centers on who has it worst, where improvement is treated with suspicion, where medical advice flows freely from people with no medical training, and where your entire identity gradually narrows to "sick person." You log off feeling worse than when you logged on.

Learn to tell the difference. If a group makes you feel hopeless more often than hopeful, leave it. If someone online tells you to try a treatment that your doctor has not recommended, do not act on it without talking to your medical team first. If you notice that you are spending more time reading about your conditions than living your life, that is a signal to step back.

Fear of missing out is a specific kind of pain for teens with chronic illness. You open your phone and see your friends at a concert, at a party, at a football game, doing all the things your body will not let you do today. That feeling is not silly. It is grief, small and sharp, and it comes back every time.

What helps is not pretending you do not care. What helps is building a life that has good things in it even on the days you cannot leave the house. A video call with a friend who makes you laugh. A show you are watching with someone. A hobby that does not require standing. A text thread that makes you feel included. The goal is not to replace what you are missing. The goal is to make sure your life has enough in it that the missing does not swallow everything else.

Action Step: This week, send one message to one person your age who has a similar condition. It can be someone from an online group, a classmate, or a friend of a friend. The message can be as simple as "Hey, I have POTS too. How are you doing with it?" One connection can change more than you think.

Your Mind and Your Body Are on the Same Team

Here is something that probably nobody has explained to you clearly: anxiety that comes from POTS is not the same as anxiety disorder.

When your autonomic nervous system dumps adrenaline into your bloodstream because you stood up, your body produces the exact same physical sensations as a panic attack: racing heart, shallow breathing, dizziness, trembling, a feeling of dread. Your brain, receiving these signals, does what any brain would do. It concludes that something is wrong and tells you to be afraid.

This is not an anxiety disorder. This is your nervous system misfiring and your brain responding logically to bad information. The distinction matters because the treatment is different. Anxiety disorder responds to therapy and sometimes medication that targets the brain. POTS-driven anxiety responds to POTS treatment: fluids, salt, compression, exercise, and medications that stabilize your heart rate and blood pressure. If a doctor has told you "it is just anxiety" without evaluating you for dysautonomia, the anxiety diagnosis may be incomplete.

That said, living with chronic illness during your teenage years can absolutely cause real anxiety and real depression that go beyond the physiological effects of the conditions themselves. If you are feeling persistently sad, withdrawn, hopeless, or unable to enjoy things you used to love, those feelings deserve attention. Not because they prove you are weak, but because they prove you are human and your situation is hard.

Finding a therapist who understands chronic illness makes a significant difference. A therapist who does not understand the trifecta might accidentally reinforce the message that your physical symptoms are caused by your emotions, which puts you back in the same box you have been fighting to escape. Look for therapists who list chronic illness, chronic pain, or medical conditions in their specialties. Ask in your first session: "How do you approach therapy for someone whose physical symptoms are caused by diagnosed medical conditions, not by psychological distress?" Their answer will tell you quickly if they are the right fit.

Grief is another emotion that deserves a name. You may be grieving the version of your teenage years you expected to have. The sports seasons, the late nights, the spontaneous road trips, the ability to stand in line for a concert without calculating the cost. That grief is legitimate.

It does not mean you are ungrateful for what you do have. It means you are honest about what was taken.

Pacing is a skill that can protect both your body and your mind. The concept is simple: instead of doing everything on good days and collapsing on bad days, spread your energy more evenly across the week. Think of your energy as a daily budget. You start each day with a set amount (some days more, some days less). Every activity costs something: getting dressed, going to school, walking between classes, paying attention in class, socializing, homework. If you spend your entire budget by noon, you will have nothing left for the afternoon.

Learning to pace takes practice. It means saying no to a second social event in one day even when you want to go. It means resting before you feel exhausted, not after. It means accepting that doing less now often means you can do more over the course of a week than if you push through and crash.

Oscar discovered pacing after a particularly bad boom-and-bust cycle during his junior year. He attended a full day of school on Monday, pushed through a basketball game on Tuesday, and spent Wednesday through Friday in bed. His physical therapist helped him see the pattern. "You are treating your energy like a credit card," she said. "You keep borrowing from tomorrow, and tomorrow keeps coming with a bigger bill." Oscar started budgeting his energy the way he budgeted his money: with a plan, a limit, and the understanding that running out had consequences.

Action Step: Tonight, write down everything you did today and estimate how much energy each activity cost on a scale of 1 to 5. Look at where you spent the most. Ask yourself: was there one thing I could have shortened or skipped to have energy left for something I actually wanted to do? That is the beginning of pacing.

Summary

Your symptoms have biological explanations. POTS, EDS, and MCAS are real, measurable medical conditions. The inconsistency of your symptoms is a feature of these diseases, not evidence against them.

You control who gets your story. Some people earn the full explanation. Some get the short version. Some get nothing. That is your right.

Online communities can be powerful support or slow poison. Choose groups that make you feel less alone and more capable, not groups that make your illness your entire identity.

Anxiety driven by dysautonomia is different from anxiety disorder, and the treatments are different too. Real depression and grief can also accompany chronic illness and deserve professional support from a therapist who understands medical conditions.

Pacing is the skill that protects everything else. Budget your energy the way you budget money: with awareness, limits, and the understanding that overdrawing today means paying for it tomorrow.

You did not choose these conditions. But you get to choose how you respond to them. And the fact that you are reading this book, learning about your body, and looking for ways to manage your life tells me that you are already responding with more strength than you probably give yourself credit for.

Chapter 13 Keep Your Social Life Alive

Lucia had 847 followers on Instagram and zero people she could call at midnight when she could not sleep because her heart rate would not drop below 110.

She had been popular before the trifecta. Volleyball team, drama club, a group of six girls who ate lunch together every day and spent weekends at each other's houses. Then the absences started. First a few days. Then weeks. Then stretches where she was gone so long that when she came back, the lunch table conversations had moved on to people and events she knew nothing about.

Nobody was cruel about it. Nobody told her to go away. It was worse than that. They were polite. They smiled and said "Hey, Lucia" and made room for her, and then continued talking about things she had not been there for. She sat at the edge of a circle that had closed without her.

By sophomore year, Lucia had stopped trying. She ate lunch in the library. She told her mother she preferred it that way. Her mother did not believe her, and she was right not to.

Chronic illness does not just steal your health. It steals your social life, quietly, one missed hangout at a time. The people who leave are not always bad people. They are teenagers who do not know how to handle a friend whose body does something they cannot see or understand. They drift. And you, stuck at home or stuck in the nurse's office, drift too.

This chapter is about stopping that drift. Not by pretending you can keep up with the pace of healthy teenage life (you cannot, and trying will make you sicker), but by building a social life that works with your body instead of demanding things your body cannot give.

Stay Connected Without Burning Out

Friendship when you are chronically ill requires a different strategy than friendship when you are healthy. The old model, where you prove your loyalty by showing up to everything, staying late, and being available on demand, does not work anymore. You need a new model, one based on consistency over intensity.

A ten-minute phone call twice a week builds a stronger friendship than one epic hangout followed by three weeks of silence while you recover. A daily text thread where you and a friend share small, funny observations keeps you in each other's lives even when you cannot be in the same room. A standing virtual movie night, where you and a friend press play at the same time and text reactions back and forth, creates a shared experience without requiring you to leave your bed.

The key is regularity. People stay connected through repetition, not drama. Small, predictable points of contact matter more than grand gestures.

When you do have energy for in-person time, use it wisely. Invite a friend to your house for a low-key hangout rather than meeting at a loud restaurant. Choose activities where you can sit or lie down comfortably: watching something together, cooking (if your MCAS allows it), playing a game, working on a project side by side. Save your energy for the person, not the activity.

Gabriel found that his friendships improved when he stopped apologizing for his limitations and started making specific plans instead. Instead of "Sorry I cannot hang out, I am sick again," he started saying, "I am having a rough week, but I could do a video call on Thursday evening. Want to watch that show together?" The shift from cancellation to invitation changed the tone of every conversation.

When someone says "but you do not look sick," the temptation is to justify, explain, and prove. Resist it. The most effective response is calm and brief. "These conditions are internal. They do not show on the outside, but they affect how I feel and what I can do. Thanks for understanding." Then change the subject. You do not need to convince anyone. You need to conserve your energy for the people who already believe you.

Here is the harder truth about friendships during chronic illness: some will not survive. Not because those people are terrible, but because teenage friendships often depend on shared daily experience, and when you are absent for weeks at a time, the shared experience shrinks. This loss hurts. It is okay to feel that hurt without turning it into a story about being abandoned or unlovable. People grow apart for all kinds of reasons. Illness just accelerates a process that happens naturally to many friendships during the high school years.

The friends who stay are the ones worth investing in. They are the ones who text you on your bad days without expecting a response. They are the ones who visit even when all you can do is lie on the couch. They are the ones who learned what POTS means because you matter enough for them to look it up. Those friendships may be fewer in number than what you had before. They are usually deeper in quality.

Coralie lost most of her friend group during sophomore year when her MCAS flares kept her homebound for weeks at a time. By junior year, she had two close friends instead of ten. "I used to think having fewer friends meant I was failing at being a teenager," she said. "Now I think having two people who actually know me is worth more than a crowded lunch table where nobody notices when I am gone."

Action Step: Choose one friend you have been losing touch with. Send them a specific, low-pressure invitation this week: "Want to video call Wednesday after dinner?" or "Can you come over Saturday afternoon? We could just hang out and watch something." Specific beats vague. Easy beats ambitious.

Date on Your Terms

Dating with chronic illness brings up questions that your healthy friends never have to consider. When do you tell someone about your conditions? How much do you share? What happens when a date involves standing in a long line, eating at a restaurant with MCAS triggers, or going to a concert where the crowd and the heat could make you faint?

There is no perfect timeline for disclosure. Some teens prefer to mention their conditions early, before a first date, so that the other person knows what they are getting into. Others prefer to wait until they have a sense of the person's character, sharing after a few conversations but before anything too physical or logistically complicated.

What matters more than timing is tone. If you treat your conditions as shameful secrets, the other person will pick up on that energy. If you mention them calmly and practically, the way you might mention a food preference or a schedule conflict, the conversation tends to go better. "I have some health conditions that affect my energy and what I can eat. It is not a big deal most of the time, but I wanted you to know so we can plan around it." That is enough for an early conversation.

Margot had a first date at a coffee shop. She ordered herbal tea (caffeine worsened her POTS) and told the boy across the table, matter-of-factly, that she had a heart condition that made her dizzy sometimes. He asked a few questions. She answered honestly. He said, "Okay, good to know. Want to sit outside or is it too warm?" That simple response told Margot everything she needed to know about him. He listened, he did not panic, and he adjusted without making it weird.

Pay attention to how someone responds to your conditions. A good partner accommodates: they suggest seated activities, they check the restaurant menu for safe options, they notice when you are getting tired before you say so, and they do not pressure you to keep going when your body says stop. A controlling partner uses your conditions against you: they make decisions "for your own good" without asking what you want, they use your limitations to isolate you from friends, or they guilt you for needing rest.

The difference between caring and controlling can be subtle when you are young. If you are unsure, ask yourself one question: does this person make me feel more capable or less capable? A good partner makes you feel like you can manage your life with support. A harmful partner makes you feel like you cannot manage anything without them.

Plan Social Events Like a Strategist

Prom. Concerts. Football games. Parties. School dances. Amusement parks. These events are the currency of teenage social life, and every one of them is a potential minefield for the trifecta body.

You do not have to skip them all. But you do have to plan them.

The half-day strategy works for most social events. Instead of committing to the full experience (prom from 7 p.m. to midnight, a concert from gates-open to encore), commit to the best part and leave before your body forces you to. Arrive at prom for dinner and the first hour of dancing, then have a ride home arranged. Go to the concert for the headliner and skip the opening act. Attend the first half of the football game from a seat near an exit. You will have the experience and the photos and the memory, without the three-day crash that follows pushing past your limit.

Pre-planning makes spontaneity possible, which sounds contradictory but is not. If you know in advance that you have a ride home at any time, that you have water and salt tablets in your bag, that you have antihistamines if you start flushing, and that your friend knows to help you find a place to sit if you get dizzy, then you can relax and enjoy the event instead of spending the entire time worrying about what might go wrong.

Exit strategies should feel normal, not dramatic. "I have to head out, my ride is here" works better than "I need to leave because of my medical conditions." If you plan the exit in advance and communicate it casually, nobody notices and nobody asks questions.

Felix and his friend Martin worked out a system for parties. If Felix sent Martin a specific text (just the number "5"), it meant "I need to leave in five minutes." Martin would casually say, "Hey, we should head out, I told my mom I would be home by ten," and they would leave together. Nobody at the party knew the system. Felix never had to explain his conditions in a crowded living room. And Martin never minded being the exit excuse, because good friends understand that this is what friends do.

Action Step: Think about the next social event on your calendar. Write down three things: your arrival plan, your exit plan, and the supplies you need in your bag (water, electrolytes, medications, snacks, a phone charger). Share the exit plan with one trusted person who will be there. Then go. Enjoy the parts you can. Leave before the crash.

Summary

Chronic illness steals social life through slow drift, not sudden rejection. Friends do not usually leave out of cruelty. They leave because they do not know how to stay connected to someone who is often absent.

Consistency beats intensity. Small, regular points of contact (calls, texts, virtual hangouts) build stronger friendships than rare, exhausting outings.

Dating works best when you disclose your conditions calmly and early enough for the other person to show you who they are. Watch for partners who accommodate versus those who control. The question to ask is: does this person make me feel more capable or less?

Social events do not require all-or-nothing decisions. The half-day strategy, pre-planning, and quiet exit systems let you participate in teenage life without paying for it with days of recovery.

Your social life is not over. It looks different. And different, with the right strategies, can still be good.

Chapter 14 Find What Lights You Up

Noemi was a dancer. Not a "took lessons for two years" dancer. A serious dancer. Competitive team since age nine. Six days a week of rehearsal. Trophies in a glass case in the living room. A plan to audition for a performing arts high school.

At thirteen, POTS and EDS ended all of it in the span of one semester.

It started with her knees. Subluxations during rehearsal that she pushed through until she could not. Then the dizziness, which hit hardest during turns and lifts. Then a full syncope episode during a competition warm-up that ended with her on the floor of a gymnasium and an ambulance outside. Her cardiologist pulled her from dance indefinitely. Her physical therapist confirmed what she already knew: the joint instability and the autonomic dysfunction made competitive dance too dangerous.

Noemi grieved. She cried in the car after the appointment and did not speak to her mother for the rest of the drive. She unfollowed her team's Instagram because seeing rehearsal videos felt like looking at photos of someone who had died. She told her therapist she did not know who she was anymore.

"I was a dancer," she said. "Now I am just sick."

That sentence contained the mistake and the truth at the same time. Noemi had lost something real. The grief was legitimate, and it deserved to be felt. But the conclusion she drew from it, that her identity had been erased along with her activity, was where the story needed to change.

If you have lost a sport, an activity, or a physical ability to the trifecta, this chapter is about finding what comes next. Not a replacement (nothing replaces the thing you loved), but a new source of purpose, pride, and identity that works with the body you have now.

Let Yourself Grieve Before You Rebuild

The first thing to know is that losing an athletic or creative identity during adolescence is a real loss, and it deserves real grief. You are not being dramatic. You are not overreacting. For many teens, sports and activities are not hobbies. They are communities, identities, daily structures, college plans, and sources of self-worth. Losing them is losing a version of yourself.

The mistake some well-meaning adults make is rushing past the grief. "You will find something else." "At least you still have school." "There are more important things than sports." These statements are technically true and emotionally useless. They skip the part where you get to be sad about what happened.

Give yourself time to feel the loss. Talk about it with someone who listens without fixing (a friend, a therapist, a parent who can sit with your sadness instead of trying to solve it). Write about it if that helps. Be angry if you need to be. The feelings are not the problem. Getting stuck in the feelings permanently is the problem. And the best way to avoid getting stuck is to let the feelings move through rather than trying to lock them down.

Sebastian lost baseball in tenth grade when his EDS worsened to the point where his shoulder dislocated every time he threw overhand. His coach suggested he could still help by keeping stats in the dugout. Sebastian tried it for one game and left at the fourth inning. "Being in the dugout was worse than being at home," he said later. "At home I could pretend I was just busy. In the dugout, I had to watch everyone doing the thing I could not do anymore."

Sebastian's reaction was not weakness. It was a healthy recognition that the dugout was a setting that sharpened his grief rather than helping it heal. Sometimes the bridge back to involvement in a former activity works. Sometimes it does not. You get to decide which.

What nobody tells you about athletic identity loss is that it can affect how you see yourself in ways that go beyond the sport. If you were the fast kid, the strong kid, the kid who scored the winning goal, that identity shaped how you walked into a room. It shaped how you introduced yourself. It shaped your confidence. Losing the activity can feel like losing the confidence that came with it, because for years the two were welded together.

The work of rebuilding identity is separating who you are from what you could do. You were never just a dancer, a baseball player, a swimmer. You were a person who happened to be good at those things. The qualities that made you good at them (discipline, competitiveness, willingness to practice, love of teamwork) did not vanish when the activity did. Those qualities are portable. They are waiting for a new place to land.

Discover Activities That Fit Your Body Now

The goal is not to find an activity that makes you forget about the one you lost. The goal is to find something that gives you the same things the old activity gave you: a sense of progress, a community, a reason to work at something, and a feeling of accomplishment.

For some teens, that means adapting the physical activity to fit the trifecta body. Swimming in a temperature-controlled pool is one of the safest and most effective exercises for POTS, EDS, and MCAS combined, as we discussed in Chapter 7. The water supports your joints, provides natural compression against blood pooling, and eliminates heat as a mast cell activator (if the pool temperature is properly managed). Recumbent cycling puts no stress on unstable joints and keeps the heart rate in a manageable range. Yoga, with modifications for hypermobility (no pushing joints past neutral, no hot yoga, no inversions that worsen POTS), can build strength and body awareness.

For other teens, the answer is not physical activity at all. It is something else entirely.

Eloise lost track and field to her POTS. She spent two months being miserable about it. Then her English teacher suggested she submit a short story to the school literary magazine. Eloise had always liked writing but had never taken it seriously because her schedule was full of practice. With the practice hours suddenly empty, she started filling them with words. By the end of junior year she had won a regional writing contest, been accepted as an editor of the literary magazine, and started a blog about living with chronic illness that had 3,000 readers. "Running gave me adrenaline," she said. "Writing gives me something I did not know I needed. It gives me a voice."

Creative pursuits (writing, visual art, music that does not strain hypermobile joints, photography, digital design, coding, filmmaking) accommodate fluctuating energy because they can be done sitting or lying down, paused and resumed, and adjusted to match how you feel on any given day. They also produce something tangible that represents your effort and growth, which matters when your body keeps telling you that you cannot do things.

Academic competitions (debate, Model UN, Science Olympiad, math league, quiz bowl) offer the competitive rush and team identity that sports provided, often with less physical demand. If brain fog is a barrier, look for events where you can prepare in advance rather than performing under live, timed pressure.

Clubs and organizations that center on a cause rather than a skill (student government, volunteering, advocacy work, peer mentoring) let you contribute meaningfully even when your energy fluctuates. You can write a speech from bed. You can plan an event over email. You can mentor a younger student by phone.

Action Step: Make a list of three things you enjoyed about your old activity. Not the activity itself, but the feeling it gave you. Was it competition? Community? Physical release? Creative expression? A sense of getting better at something over time? Now brainstorm three new activities that might provide those same feelings within the limits your body sets today. Try one this month.

Push for Programs That Include You

If your school does not offer adaptive PE options, modified sports participation, or inclusive extracurricular policies, you have the right to ask for them. As we discussed in Chapter 9, your 504 plan or IEP can include provisions for modified PE and alternative activity credit. But sometimes the change needs to go beyond your individual plan.

Adaptive sports programs are growing but remain unevenly distributed. Some communities have adaptive swimming teams, wheelchair basketball leagues, seated volleyball programs, and inclusive yoga classes. Others have nothing. Check with your local parks and recreation department, YMCA or YWCA, adaptive sports organizations, and disability resource centers at nearby colleges.

If nothing is available in your area, consider becoming the person who starts something. It sounds like a big ask, and it is. But teens with chronic illness have started adaptive fitness clubs at their schools, organized inclusive intramural leagues, and petitioned athletic departments to create modified participation tracks. These efforts take energy, and you should only take them on if you have it to spare. But the impact extends beyond you. The next kid at your school who gets diagnosed with the trifecta will find a program already waiting.

Advocacy itself can become a meaningful activity. Writing about your experience (for a school paper, a blog, or a condition-specific organization), speaking at school assemblies about invisible illness, or mentoring newly diagnosed teens through online support groups all provide purpose, community, and the particular satisfaction of turning a painful experience into something useful. Valeria started recording short video explanations of what POTS feels like and posting them on social media. She was not trying to go viral. She was trying to help one person feel less confused. The videos reached far more than one person, and the responses from other teens who said "this is exactly what I have been trying to explain to people" gave Valeria something she had not felt since leaving her swim team: the sense that she was good at something that mattered.

Julian started an inclusive fitness club at his high school during his senior year. It met twice a week in the school gym and offered low-impact activities (stretching, light weights, recumbent bikes) alongside standard options. The club attracted not only students with chronic illness but also students who simply did not enjoy traditional PE. By its second semester, it had 24 members and a waiting list. The school added it to the official club roster the following year.

Not every teen will start a club. Not every teen should. But every teen deserves to know that the absence of a program is not the end of the conversation. It can be the beginning of one.

Summary

Losing a sport or activity to chronic illness is a real loss that deserves real grief. You are not being dramatic. You are mourning a part of your identity, and that takes time.

The rebuild starts by identifying what the old activity gave you emotionally (competition, community, expression, progress) and finding new activities that provide the same feelings within the limits your body sets.

Swimming, recumbent cycling, and modified yoga offer physical activity that supports trifecta management. Creative pursuits, academic competitions, and cause-based organizations offer identity, community, and accomplishment without requiring a body that cooperates every day.

Adaptive programs are growing but unevenly available. If your school or community does not have what you need, consider advocating for its creation, both for yourself and for the teens who come after you.

You are more than what your body can do on its best day. You are also what you build, what you create, and what you contribute, on every kind of day.

PART V TRANSITIONING TO ADULT CARE

Chapter 15 Start the Transition Early

Valeria turned 18 on a Tuesday. On Wednesday, she had a cardiology appointment. She walked into the same office she had visited since she was 14, sat in the same chair, and waited for the same nurse to call her name. Everything felt normal until the receptionist handed her a clipboard and said, "Since you are now 18, you will need to sign your own consent forms. And we will need to update our records. Your parents can no longer access your medical information without your written permission."

Valeria looked at the forms. She did not know her insurance ID number. She could not list all of her medications without checking her phone. She did not understand what "HIPAA authorization" meant. She had never scheduled her own appointment, called in a prescription refill, or explained her medical history to anyone without her mother sitting beside her filling in the gaps.

Her mother, sitting in the waiting room, was not allowed back without Valeria's consent. For the first time in four years of managing three chronic conditions, Valeria was alone with her medical team. And she was not ready.

This scene plays out in clinics across the country every week. The legal transition to adult medical autonomy happens on a specific birthday, but the skill transition that should precede it rarely happens on any schedule at all. Research shows that the vast majority of adolescents with chronic conditions do not receive the recommended preparation for managing their own healthcare (McManus et al., 2020). They are handed adult responsibility without adult skills. The result is missed appointments, medication errors, lapsed insurance, and a dangerous gap in care during one of the most medically vulnerable periods of their lives.

The transition from pediatric to adult care is not a single event. It is a process that should begin years before your teen's 18th birthday and continue years after. This chapter lays out the timeline, the skills, and the tools that make that process work.

Build Skills in Stages

The transition works best when it is gradual, predictable, and matched to your teen's developmental readiness rather than their chronological age alone. Research suggests starting the conversation about future independence as early as age 12 to 14 and building skills progressively through high school (Got Transition, 2020).

Between ages 14 and 16, the focus is health literacy. Your teen should begin learning the names of their conditions and what each one means in plain language. They should know the names of their medications, the doses, the purpose of each, and the most common side effects. They should be able to describe their symptoms clearly enough that a new provider could understand their baseline. This is the period for learning, not doing. Your teen observes while you manage, but they start paying attention with intention.

Clara's mother started this process by having Clara read the appointment notes from every visit. "Tell me what the doctor said today, in your own words," she would say in the car on the way home. At first, Clara could barely recall the main points. By age 15, she could recount the visit accurately, name the medication changes, and explain why they were made.

Between ages 16 and 17, the focus shifts to practice. Your teen begins performing tasks with your supervision. They call to schedule their own appointments while you listen. They fill their own pill organizer. They check their own heart rate and blood pressure logs. They practice explaining their conditions to a new provider by rehearsing with you or with their current physician. They begin attending part of their appointments alone, starting with the first five minutes and gradually extending to the full visit.

Elio's cardiologist made this shift deliberately. At age 16, she started each appointment by asking Elio directly, "What has changed since our last visit?" rather than looking to his mother. If Elio struggled to answer, the doctor waited. She did not rescue him, and she gently redirected his mother when she jumped in. Within a year, Elio could run the first ten minutes of his own appointment fluently. "It felt strange at first," he said. "Like a test I had not studied for. But after a few visits, I realized I actually knew this stuff. I just had never been asked."

Between ages 17 and 18, the focus becomes transfer. Your teen takes over primary responsibility for their medical management while you shift from manager to consultant. They handle all appointment scheduling. They manage their own medication supply and refills. They know how to access their medical records through patient portals. They understand their insurance coverage well enough to know what is in-network, what requires prior authorization, and what their copay is.

After age 18, your role changes legally and practically. Your teen is now the decision-maker. You become a resource they can call when they have questions, a safety net for emergencies, and an advocate they can invite into conversations when they choose to. This shift can feel abrupt for parents who have spent years managing every aspect of their child's care. Planning for it makes the adjustment easier for everyone.

Action Step: Assess where your teen falls on this timeline right now. Can they name all of their medications and doses? Can they explain their conditions to a stranger? Can they schedule an appointment by phone? Identify the biggest gap and choose one skill to practice this month.

Teach the Skills That Clinics Assume

Healthcare systems assume that adult patients can perform a set of skills that nobody teaches in school and that many chronically ill teens have never practiced because their parents handled everything.

Understanding diagnoses means more than knowing the acronyms. Your teen should be able to explain POTS, EDS, and MCAS in two or three sentences each, clearly enough that an urgent care doctor who has never heard of these conditions can understand the basics. As we practiced in Chapter 1, the scaffolding-wiring-security system framework works well for this purpose.

Medication literacy goes beyond knowing which pills to take. Your teen should understand why each medication was chosen (what condition it treats, what symptom it addresses), what to do if they miss a dose, which medications cannot be stopped abruptly, and which over-the-counter medications to avoid (NSAIDs can worsen MCAS in some patients, for example). They should know how to call in a refill, how to handle a lapsed prescription, and how to recognize side effects that warrant contacting their provider.

Lab result literacy means knowing what the numbers mean. Tryptase levels, heart rate variability data, electrolyte panels, and complete blood counts are all part of trifecta management. Your teen does not need to interpret results at a physician's level, but they should be able to look at a lab report and know which values are flagged, what those values relate to, and what questions to ask their provider about them.

Insurance literacy is perhaps the least glamorous and most consequential skill on this list. Hugo's family discovered this when he went to an urgent care clinic during his first semester of college. He handed over his insurance card, was treated for a POTS flare, and received a bill for $1,800 three weeks later because the clinic was out-of-network. Hugo had never been taught to check network status before seeking care. His parents had always handled that.

Teach your teen to find their insurance card, identify in-network providers, understand their deductible and copay structure, and call the insurance company to verify coverage before scheduling appointments with new providers. These are not exciting skills. They are the skills that prevent financial crises during a period when medical needs do not pause.

Practice these skills while the stakes are low. Before your teen's next specialist appointment, have them call the insurance company to verify that the provider is in-network and to confirm the copay amount. Walk them through reading an Explanation of Benefits statement after a recent visit. Show them how to use the insurance company's website or app to search for in-network providers by specialty and location. Each of these exercises takes 15 minutes and builds a skill they will use hundreds of times in adulthood.

Noemi's parents turned insurance education into a monthly dinner table conversation during her junior year. Each month, they reviewed one aspect of health insurance: how deductibles work, what "prior authorization" means, why the same medication costs different amounts at different pharmacies, and what to do if a claim is denied. By the time Noemi left for college, she could handle her own insurance questions. Her roommate, who had never been taught any of this, was still calling her mother every time she needed to fill a prescription.

Create the Portable Medical Summary

Every trifecta teen approaching the transition to adult care needs a single document that contains their complete medical picture. This document goes by different names: a medical summary, a health passport, a care transition document. Regardless of what you call it, it serves one purpose: it allows a new provider to understand your teen's full situation in under five minutes.

The portable medical summary should include the following: full legal name, date of birth, and emergency contact information; a list of all confirmed diagnoses with the date of each diagnosis; current medications with doses, frequencies, and prescribing providers; known allergies and adverse drug reactions; a list of all current specialists with names, specialties, and contact information; a brief description of the emergency protocols for each condition (what to do for syncope, dislocation, anaphylaxis); most recent lab results with dates; surgical history if relevant; and the name and contact information for the current primary care provider.

Keep this document in three places: as a digital file on your teen's phone, as a printed copy in their wallet or medical kit, and as a shared document that you and your teen can both access and update.

Martin's mother created his medical summary when he was 16 and updated it before every specialist appointment. By the time Martin started college, the document was four pages long and contained everything a new provider would need. When Martin went to the campus health center during his first week with a POTS flare, he handed the nurse the summary. She read it, looked up, and said, "This is the most helpful thing any patient has ever brought me." The summary saved Martin from having to explain three complex conditions through brain fog, on his feet, in an unfamiliar clinic.

Action Step: Sit down with your teen this weekend and start building the portable medical summary. Use the template in Appendix B of this book. Fill in what you can together, and mark the gaps that need information from your providers. Aim to have a complete first draft within one month.

Summary

The transition from pediatric to adult care is a process, not a single event. It should begin at age 14 and progress through four stages: health literacy, supervised practice, responsibility transfer, and full self-management with parental consultation.

The skills that adult healthcare systems assume patients have (diagnosis explanation, medication management, lab interpretation, insurance navigation) must be taught deliberately because no one else will teach them.

A portable medical summary is the single most useful tool for the transition. It gives new providers immediate access to your teen's full medical picture and prevents the dangerous information gaps that occur during provider changes.

Start building these skills and tools now, regardless of your teen's age. Every month of preparation before age 18 reduces the chaos after it.

Chapter 16 Find Providers Who Listen

Oscar had an excellent pediatric cardiologist. Dr. Reyes knew his POTS history from diagnosis at age 13 through stabilization at age 16. She knew which medications he had tried and failed, which dosing adjustments worked, and which symptoms indicated a flare versus a normal bad day. She spoke to his mother at every appointment. She emailed his school nurse at the beginning of each year. She was the center of his medical world.

When Oscar turned 19, Dr. Reyes told him it was time to transition to an adult cardiologist. She gave him three names. Oscar's mother called the first one. The office said the earliest available appointment was four months away. She called the second. That office did not accept Oscar's insurance. She called the third. The receptionist paused and said, "We do not really see patients for POTS here. You might want to try a neurologist."

Oscar did not see a cardiologist for seven months. During that time, his fludrocortisone prescription lapsed because the new pharmacy needed a prescribing provider, and he did not have one. His POTS symptoms returned with a severity he had not experienced in three years. By the time his mother found an adult cardiologist who understood the condition, Oscar had missed a semester of college.

This story repeats in families across the country. The transition from pediatric to adult care is not just an emotional shift. It is a structural problem. Pediatric providers who specialize in the trifecta are rare. Adult providers who understand pediatric-onset presentations of these conditions are even rarer. The gap between the two systems can swallow months of progress.

This chapter will help you find adult providers who understand the trifecta, vet them before committing, and build a care team that can carry your teen forward.

Understand Why Adult Care Feels Different

The shift from pediatric to adult medicine is not just a change of doctor. It is a change of culture. Understanding the differences in advance helps families adjust without feeling blindsided.

Pediatric care is family-centered. Parents are expected at appointments. Communication flows between the provider, the teen, and the parent as a unit. The provider often coordinates across specialties, checks in proactively, and frames care in the context of the child's school life, development, and family situation.

Adult care is individual-centered. The patient is the primary point of contact. Parents may or may not be in the room, depending on the patient's preference and HIPAA authorization. Communication between specialists is less coordinated, and the patient is expected to manage their own referrals, follow-ups, and information flow. The provider focuses on the disease, not the life circumstances surrounding it.

Neither model is wrong. But the shift can feel like a loss, especially for families who have spent years building relationships within the pediatric system. A meta-ethnography of youth experiences during this transition found that young people consistently described feeling unprepared, unsupported, and forced to manage new activities on their own, characterizing themselves as "expert novices" who had knowledge but lacked the skills to apply it independently .

Paloma described the difference this way: "My pediatric cardiologist asked about my school, my friends, my sleep. She knew I was in debate club. My adult cardiologist looks at my heart rate numbers, adjusts my meds, and asks if I have any questions. The appointment lasts 12 minutes. It is efficient, but it does not feel like anyone is taking care of me." Paloma's feeling is common and worth naming. The warmth of pediatric care is not something adult care replaces. It is something you learn to provide for yourself, through the self-advocacy skills you have been building throughout this book and through the relationships you cultivate with your adult providers over time.

Some young adults find that the adult care model actually suits them better once they adjust. The independence can feel respectful rather than cold. The efficiency can feel like trust rather than dismissal. Marcel, who had sometimes felt patronized by the family-centered approach of pediatric care, appreciated that his adult providers spoke directly to him without looking to his mother for confirmation. "For the first time, I felt like the expert on my own body," he said. "That was uncomfortable for about two appointments. Then it felt right."

The culture gap widens when the adult provider is unfamiliar with the trifecta. A pediatric cardiologist who sees 50 POTS patients a year understands the condition deeply. An adult cardiologist who has seen three POTS patients in their career may default to treatments appropriate for other forms of tachycardia, dismiss the severity of symptoms, or suggest that the patient has "outgrown" the condition because some adolescent POTS patients improve by their early twenties.

Specialty mapping helps families plan the transition. Your pediatric cardiologist will likely hand off to an adult cardiologist or an electrophysiologist with autonomic dysfunction experience. Your geneticist may continue to follow your teen into adulthood (genetics does not have a strict pediatric cutoff) or may refer to an adult rheumatologist for ongoing EDS management. Your pediatric allergist/immunologist will refer to an adult allergist or an internist with mast cell disease experience. Your coordinating primary care physician may change if your teen moves for college or work, making it important to establish adult primary care in the new location early.

Vet Providers Before You Commit

Not every provider who accepts patients with POTS, EDS, or MCAS actually understands these conditions. Vetting before scheduling saves time, money, and the emotional cost of starting over with someone who is not the right fit.

Before the first appointment, call the office and ask direct questions. "Does this provider have experience treating patients with postural orthostatic tachycardia syndrome?" is a better question than "Do you treat heart conditions?" If the receptionist does not know, ask to speak with a nurse or physician assistant. A practice that cannot answer this question at all is unlikely to have the expertise your teen needs.

Ask about the provider's approach to multisystem conditions. A cardiologist who treats POTS as an isolated heart rate problem without considering the EDS and MCAS connections will provide fragmented care. The ideal adult provider recognizes the trifecta pattern and understands that treatment decisions for one condition affect the others, as we discussed in Chapter 7.

Red flags that a provider is not the right fit include dismissing symptoms as anxiety without evaluation, stating that POTS is something patients "grow out of" (some do improve, but many do not, and dismissal is different from honest prognostic discussion), being unwilling to coordinate with other specialists, and expressing skepticism about MCAS as a diagnosis.

The overlapping appointment strategy can ease the transition significantly. Rather than a hard cutoff where your teen sees the pediatric provider one month and the adult provider the next, arrange a period of overlap where both are involved. Some pediatric practices will continue seeing a patient for six to 12 months after the formal transition while the adult provider gets up to speed. During this window, the pediatric provider can answer the adult provider's questions, confirm baseline histories, and provide continuity for the patient.

Eloise's pediatric cardiologist scheduled a phone call with her new adult electrophysiologist before Eloise's first adult appointment. They discussed her medication history, her exercise tolerance, her most effective treatment combination, and the patterns of her flares. When Eloise walked into the new office, the adult provider already knew her case. "Dr. Reyes told me about your situation," he said. "Let us pick up where she left off." That single phone call eliminated months of re-establishing context.

Action Step: If your teen is within two years of transitioning, ask the current pediatric specialist for adult provider recommendations now. Request at least three names. Call each office and ask: "Does this provider have specific experience with POTS (or EDS, or MCAS)? How many patients with this condition does the provider currently manage?" The answers will tell you where to start.

Build a Hybrid Team With Telehealth

The shortage of trifecta-experienced providers is real, and it is not limited to any one region. Many families drive two, four, or six hours to see the right specialist. For young adults who have moved away for college or work, maintaining access to experienced providers requires creative solutions.

Telehealth has expanded access significantly. Many POTS, EDS, and MCAS specialists now offer virtual consultations for follow-up visits, medication management, and second opinions. A teen who lives in a small town can see a trifecta-experienced cardiologist in a major medical center without traveling, as long as the provider is licensed in the patient's state.

The hybrid care model pairs a local primary care provider who handles day-to-day management (prescription refills, urgent issues, basic labs) with a remote specialist who guides the treatment plan through periodic telehealth visits. The local provider follows the specialist's recommendations and escalates when something falls outside their comfort zone. The specialist reviews records, adjusts the care plan, and is available for consultation when the local provider has questions.

State licensing limitations remain a barrier. A physician licensed only in California cannot legally treat a patient located in Texas via telehealth, even if that patient was previously seen in person in California. Some states have reciprocity agreements. Interstate medical licensure compacts have expanded options, but coverage is not universal. Before relying on telehealth, confirm that the specialist is licensed in your teen's state of residence, or that an exception applies.

Some specialized clinics have responded to this problem by obtaining licensure in multiple states specifically to serve their chronic illness patient populations. The EDS Clinic, for example, operates across more than a dozen states through a combination of in-person and virtual appointments. Ask any potential telehealth specialist which states they are licensed in before scheduling, and verify that your teen's current location is covered.

Provider directories maintained by Dysautonomia International, the Ehlers-Danlos Society, and the Mast Cell Disease Society can help identify specialists who see patients in your teen's area, either in person or by telehealth. These directories are not endorsements, and the quality of individual providers still needs to be verified, but they offer a starting point that is far better than cold-calling random cardiologists from an insurance company's provider list.

Gabriel's family built a hybrid team when he left for college 300 miles from home. His local adult primary care provider in the college town handled his prescriptions, monthly vitals, and routine blood work. His POTS specialist back home conducted telehealth visits every three months to review his data, adjust medications, and coordinate with the local provider. His EDS physical therapist was local to the college. His MCAS allergist remained the same, seen during school breaks and by phone between visits. The system was not perfect, but it kept Gabriel connected to experienced providers while building a local safety net.

Summary

Adult providers who understand pediatric-onset trifecta presentations are rare, and finding them requires active effort. Do not wait until the transition is upon you to start searching.

The culture shift from family-centered pediatric care to individual-centered adult care is significant. Young adults describe feeling like "expert novices" during this transition. Understanding the differences in advance reduces the shock.

Vet providers before committing by asking specific questions about their experience with POTS, EDS, and MCAS. Use the overlapping appointment strategy to ensure continuity, and ask the pediatric provider to communicate directly with the new adult provider.

Telehealth and hybrid care models can bridge the specialist gap for young adults who have moved away from their pediatric medical team. Pair a local primary care provider with a remote specialist to maintain both access and safety.

The best time to build the adult care team is before you need it. Start now.

Chapter 17 Handle the Legal and Financial Shift

On the morning of his 18th birthday, Sebastian's mother called his allergist's office to ask about a medication change. The receptionist said, "I am sorry, but we cannot discuss Sebastian's care with you without his written authorization on file."

Sebastian's mother had managed his MCAS medications for five years. She knew his tryptase levels, his antihistamine rotation schedule, and the exact brand of epinephrine auto-injector his insurance covered. She had called this office dozens of times. And now, on the strength of a single calendar date, she was locked out.

She was not angry at the office. They were following the law. She was angry at herself for not preparing for this moment, even though she had known it was coming. HIPAA protections activate at age 18 in most states. A parent who was the primary medical advocate on Monday has no legal access to their child's records on Tuesday unless the young adult has signed specific authorization forms.

The legal and financial landscape shifts significantly when your teen turns 18. This chapter covers the three areas where that shift matters most: medical decision-making authority, insurance coverage, and disability benefits. Each area has specific steps you can take now to prevent the disruptions that catch unprepared families off guard.

Understand What Changes at 18

At age 18, your teen becomes a legal adult with full authority over their medical decisions. This means they consent to their own treatment, control access to their own medical records, and can refuse care that you believe they need. No provider can share information with you without your teen's written permission.

For families managing the trifecta, this transition has practical consequences that go beyond philosophy. If your teen has brain fog from POTS that impairs their decision-making on some days, they are still the legal decision-maker. If your teen is in the ER during a severe MCAS flare and cannot communicate clearly, you may not be able to access their records or speak to the treating physician without authorization on file.

Two documents can preserve parental involvement without overriding the young adult's autonomy. A HIPAA authorization form, signed by your teen, gives you permission to access their medical records and speak with their providers. This form should list every provider and facility your teen sees, and it should be updated annually or whenever the provider list changes. Many families complete this form the week of the teen's 18th birthday and file copies with every provider.

A healthcare power of attorney (sometimes called a healthcare proxy or advance directive) designates someone to make medical decisions on the young adult's behalf if they become unable to make decisions for themselves. This is not the same as the HIPAA authorization. The HIPAA form allows information sharing. The healthcare power of attorney allows decision-making during incapacity. For a trifecta teen who may experience severe brain fog, syncope, or anaphylaxis, having this document in place provides a critical safety net.

These forms are simple to complete but easy to forget. Many families intend to handle them "at some point" and then never do, until a crisis makes the absence painfully clear. Do not wait for the crisis. Treat these forms with the same urgency as filling a prescription or scheduling an appointment. They take 20 minutes to complete and can be the difference between a coordinated emergency response and chaos.

Felix's family completed both documents on his 18th birthday. His mother kept copies in a folder, uploaded them to a shared cloud drive, and filed originals with his primary care provider, his cardiologist, and the local emergency room. Three months later, when Felix was admitted to the ER during a severe MCAS flare and was too disoriented to explain his medication list, his mother pulled up the documents on her phone and was able to consult with the treating physician within minutes. Without those forms, she would have been standing in the hallway while a doctor who had never heard of MCAS made treatment decisions alone.

Action Step: Before your teen turns 18 (or immediately if they have already turned 18), complete a HIPAA authorization form and a healthcare power of attorney. Many hospitals and medical practices offer free templates. Your teen's pediatrician can often provide both forms at a routine visit. File copies with every provider on the team.

Plan the Insurance Transition

Under the Affordable Care Act, young adults can remain on a parent's health insurance plan until age 26, regardless of student status, marital status, or financial independence. This provision has been one of the most significant protections for young adults with chronic illness, and it buys time during the transition period.

But remaining on a parent's plan does not mean the coverage remains unchanged. If your teen moves to a different state for college or work, the parent's plan may have a limited network in the new location. Out-of-network care costs more, sometimes dramatically more, as Hugo's family discovered during his urgent care visit in Chapter 15. Before your teen moves, check the plan's network coverage in the new location and identify in-network providers for each specialty.

Medicaid eligibility is available for young adults with disabilities whose income and assets fall below state-specific thresholds. Supplemental Security Income (SSI) recipients are automatically eligible for Medicaid in most states. For trifecta young adults who are unable to work or who work part-time due to their conditions, Medicaid can provide coverage for medications, specialist visits, and therapies that private insurance may not fully cover.

College student health plans are another option, but they vary widely in quality. Some are robust enough to cover specialist visits, prescription medications, and emergency care. Others are bare-bones plans that cover campus health center visits and little else. Before enrolling your teen in a student health plan, compare the coverage to the parent's plan. Look specifically at the formulary (does it cover your teen's specific medications?), the specialist network (are there trifecta-experienced providers in-network?), and the out-of-pocket maximums.

When the parent's plan expires at age 26, or if your teen loses access to parental insurance sooner, the options include employer-sponsored insurance, ACA marketplace plans, and Medicaid. Each has its own enrollment periods, eligibility requirements, and coverage gaps. Plan for this transition at least six months in advance.

The open enrollment period for ACA marketplace plans typically runs from November to January for coverage beginning the following year. Missing this window means waiting an entire year unless you qualify for a special enrollment period (losing other coverage, moving, or getting married can all trigger special enrollment eligibility). For a young adult with the trifecta, even a single month without insurance coverage can result in thousands of dollars in out-of-pocket medication costs and missed specialist appointments. Do not let the enrollment deadline surprise you.

Margot's family created an insurance transition timeline when she was 17. They mapped every coverage change point from age 18 through 26: when she would start college and need in-network providers near campus, when she would age off the family dental plan (a separate timeline from medical), when she would need to evaluate her own marketplace options, and when she would need to apply for Medicaid if her income remained low. Having the timeline prevented every coverage gap that caught her friends' families by surprise.

Know Your Disability Benefits Options

For young adults whose trifecta conditions prevent or significantly limit their ability to work, federal disability benefits may be available. The two primary programs are Supplemental Security Income (SSI) and Social Security Disability Insurance (SSDI).

SSI is a needs-based program for disabled individuals with limited income and assets. Young adults who have not worked enough to qualify for SSDI (which requires a work history) may qualify for SSI based on the severity of their conditions and their financial situation. Monthly SSI payments are modest (the federal base rate was $943 per month in 2024), but the program also provides automatic Medicaid eligibility in most states, which can cover the substantial medical costs of trifecta management.

The application process is notoriously complex and has a high initial denial rate. Approximately 65% of initial SSI/SSDI applications are denied, and many of those are ultimately approved on appeal (Social Security Administration, 2023). Detailed medical documentation is critical. The application should include letters from all treating specialists describing the functional limitations caused by each condition, evidence of how the conditions affect the ability to work (standing tolerance, cognitive function, unpredictable flares), and a history of treatment attempts and their outcomes.

Vocational rehabilitation services, administered by each state, can help young adults with disabilities prepare for and find employment. Services may include career counseling, job training, assistive technology, job placement assistance, and ongoing support after employment begins. For a trifecta young adult who can work but needs accommodations or a non-traditional work arrangement, vocational rehabilitation can bridge the gap between disability and employment.

The application process for vocational rehabilitation starts with your state's vocational rehabilitation agency (the name varies by state). A counselor is assigned who evaluates the young adult's abilities, limitations, and employment goals, then develops an Individualized Plan for Employment (IPE) that outlines the services needed to reach those goals. Services are provided at no cost to the individual.

Julian connected with his state's vocational rehabilitation program during his senior year of high school. His counselor helped him identify that his strengths in writing and analysis could lead to careers in research, editing, or communications, fields that offered remote work options and flexible schedules. The program funded a summer internship at a nonprofit organization that allowed him to test his tolerance for part-time work before committing to a full-time role. The internship confirmed that Julian could sustain 25 hours a week with rest breaks built into his schedule, information that shaped his job search after graduation.

Disability scholarships and financial aid are available from numerous private foundations, condition-specific organizations, and colleges. The Ehlers-Danlos Society, Dysautonomia International, and the Mast Cell Disease Society all maintain scholarship directories or award programs. Many colleges have specific scholarship funds for students with chronic illnesses or disabilities. These sources can offset the financial burden of higher education when medical expenses already strain the family budget.

The financial picture for young adults with the trifecta is rarely simple. Medical expenses, insurance costs, reduced earning capacity, and the practical costs of managing three conditions (compression garments, specialized food, supplements, copays, transportation to specialists) add up to a significant financial burden. Planning for these costs early, rather than reacting to each bill as it arrives, turns a chaotic financial situation into a manageable one.

Action Step: If your teen is approaching 18 and their conditions significantly affect their ability to work, consult with a disability benefits attorney or advocate before filing. Many offer free initial consultations. Preparation before filing dramatically improves the chance of approval and reduces the time spent in the appeals process.

Summary

At age 18, your teen gains full legal authority over their medical decisions and records. HIPAA authorization and healthcare power of attorney forms preserve parental involvement without overriding the young adult's autonomy. Complete and file these documents before or immediately at the 18th birthday.

Insurance coverage under a parent's plan can continue until age 26 under the ACA, but network limitations in new locations must be checked. Medicaid, student health plans, and marketplace options all require advance planning to avoid coverage gaps.

SSI and SSDI disability benefits are available for young adults whose trifecta conditions prevent or significantly limit work. The application process is complex with a high initial denial rate, making thorough documentation and professional guidance valuable investments.

The financial and legal systems do not pause for chronic illness. Planning ahead prevents the crises that catch unprepared families in the gap between pediatric and adult life.

Chapter 18 Build a Life That Works

Marcel left for college with three suitcases, a medical supply box, and a plan. The plan had been assembled over his senior year with input from his parents, his cardiologist, his allergist, and his physical therapist. It covered which pharmacy near campus was in-network, where to find low-histamine groceries, how to request a dorm room near the elevator, and the name of an adult cardiologist 40 minutes away who had agreed to take him on as a patient.

The plan did not cover what happened during the third week of September, when Marcel's roommate sprayed cologne in their shared bathroom and Marcel's mast cells responded with full-force flushing, hives, and throat tightness. The plan did not cover the exhaustion of walking 20 minutes across a hilly campus to each class when his POTS flared during a heat wave. The plan did not cover the loneliness of eating alone in his dorm room because the cafeteria was too loud, too warm, and served nothing he could safely eat.

Marcel called his mother on a Tuesday night and told her he wanted to come home.

She talked him through it. Not by telling him to toughen up, and not by driving there to rescue him. She helped him problem-solve. They called the disability services office together the next morning and requested a single room or a fragrance-aware roommate assignment. They emailed the dining services director about Marcel's dietary needs and arranged a meeting. They identified a campus shuttle route that would reduce his walking distance. Within two weeks, the crises were manageable and Marcel was staying.

The transition to independent living with the trifecta is not a straight line. It is a series of problems that require solutions, adjustments that require flexibility, and moments of doubt that require support. This chapter covers the practical systems that help young adults with the trifecta build lives that work, at college, at work, and on their own.

Manage College With the Trifecta

Disability services registration should happen before the first day of classes, ideally during the summer before enrollment. As we discussed in Chapter 11, the process requires documentation of diagnoses, a description of functional limitations, and specific accommodation requests. College disability services operate under different laws than K-12 schools (the ADA and Section 504 of the Rehabilitation Act, rather than IDEA), and the burden shifts to the student to request services rather than the institution to identify need.

Common college accommodations for trifecta students include priority course registration (to select classes in accessible buildings and during optimal times of day), extended time on exams, permission to record lectures, flexible attendance policies during flares, and access to a testing center with climate control and food/drink access.

Dorm accommodations can significantly affect daily health management. A single room eliminates roommate-related fragrance and allergen exposures. A ground-floor room near an elevator reduces the daily cardiovascular cost of accessing your living space. Air conditioning is not a luxury for someone with POTS and MCAS. It is a medical accommodation. A medical-grade refrigerator stores temperature-sensitive medications and allows safe food storage for low-histamine meals.

Meal plan modifications deserve early attention. Many colleges will work with students to identify safe dining options, provide ingredient information for prepared foods, or allow the student to opt out of the standard meal plan in favor of a kitchen-equipped apartment. Coralie's college allowed her to convert her meal plan to "dining dollars" that could be spent at specific food stations where she could see ingredients and avoid her triggers. The arrangement was not perfect, but it was far better than the standard buffet model.

Medication management in college requires a level of independence that many teens have not practiced. Your teen should know how to transfer prescriptions to a new pharmacy, refill medications by phone or app, store medications properly (some MCAS medications require refrigeration), and recognize when a prescription is about to run out. A weekly pill organizer, phone alarms for medication times, and a shared medication tracking app with a parent can provide scaffolding during the first year.

Medical leave is a last resort but sometimes a necessary one. If your teen's conditions destabilize to the point where attending classes is doing more harm than good, a medical withdrawal preserves their academic record and allows them to return when stable. Most colleges have specific medical leave policies, including required documentation from a physician, a defined timeline for return, and a re-enrollment process. Taking medical leave is not failure. It is strategy. Ines took a medical leave during her sophomore spring when a severe MCAS flare made attending classes impossible. She returned in the fall, finished her degree on a modified timeline, and graduated with honors.

Plan a Career That Fits Your Body

Career planning with the trifecta involves an honest assessment of what your body can and cannot sustain over the long term. This is not about lowering expectations. It is about choosing paths that let you succeed consistently rather than paths that demand a body you do not have.

Careers that accommodate fluctuating health share certain characteristics: flexible scheduling, the ability to work remotely at least some of the time, tasks that can be paused and resumed, environments that are temperature-controlled and fragrance-reduced, and low physical demand relative to cognitive demand.

Many trifecta young adults thrive in fields like writing, graphic design, software development, data analysis, counseling (virtual practice), education (with accommodations), research, and administrative roles with flexibility. Others find that creative self-employment, freelancing, or consulting allows them to control their schedule and environment in ways traditional employment does not.

Workplace accommodations under the Americans with Disabilities Act are available to qualified employees with disabilities. Common accommodations for the trifecta include a flexible or modified work schedule, the ability to work from home, a temperature-controlled workspace, a chair or standing desk appropriate for EDS, access to food and water at the workstation, and modified break schedules. Requesting accommodations requires disclosure of the disability to the employer's human resources department, but not necessarily to direct supervisors or coworkers.

Disclosure decisions in job applications and interviews are personal and strategic. You are not legally required to disclose a disability during the hiring process. The ADA prohibits employers from asking about medical conditions before making a job offer. After an offer is made, you can request accommodations and disclose only what is necessary for the accommodation to be understood. Julian's approach was to wait until he had been offered the position, then contact human resources directly: "I have a medical condition that requires a few workplace accommodations. I would like to discuss those before my start date." This framing is professional, specific, and protected by law.

Remote work has opened doors that were previously closed to many people with chronic illness. If remote work is available in your field, it may eliminate the physical toll of commuting, allow you to manage symptoms throughout the day, and let you control your environment completely. Negotiate remote work options early in the employment conversation rather than as a reactive accommodation request after problems arise.

Mateo discovered that his best work happened between 10 a.m. and 2 p.m., when his POTS symptoms were most controlled. A traditional 9-to-5 office job would have wasted his worst hours (early morning) on commuting and spent his best hours sitting in an overheated open-plan office. His remote data analysis position allowed him to start at 10, work his most demanding tasks during his peak window, take a rest break at 3, and finish lighter tasks in the evening. His productivity was higher than most of his fully healthy coworkers, because he had learned something most people never think about: when and how his body and brain worked best.

That self-knowledge, built through years of managing the trifecta, is actually a professional asset. People who have managed chronic illness since adolescence tend to be unusually skilled at planning, prioritizing, communicating clearly, solving problems under constraints, and persisting through difficulty. These are skills that employers value highly, even if they were learned in a medical context rather than a professional one.

Action Step: If your teen is beginning to think about careers, ask them to list five jobs that interest them. For each, evaluate three factors: physical demands, schedule flexibility, and remote work potential. This exercise is not about ruling options out. It is about identifying which paths naturally accommodate the trifecta and which would require significant workplace accommodation.

Prepare for Daily Living on Your Own

Independent living with the trifecta requires systems. Without systems, the daily demands of managing three conditions while also managing rent, groceries, laundry, and social life can overwhelm even a well-prepared young adult.

Medical supply management means keeping a running inventory of medications, compression garments, braces, electrolyte supplies, and emergency kit contents. Running out of a critical medication because nobody noticed the bottle was nearly empty is a preventable crisis. A simple checklist on the refrigerator, reviewed weekly, can prevent it.

Cooking with MCAS restrictions takes more planning than ordering takeout, but it gives you control over ingredients that no restaurant can match. Batch cooking on good days and freezing individual portions means that bad days do not have to mean eating food that makes you sicker. A small collection of reliable, safe recipes (maybe 10 to 15 meals you know you tolerate well) removes the daily decision burden and reduces the chance of a reaction from an unfamiliar ingredient.

Energy management in daily living, the pacing skills we discussed in Chapter 12, becomes even more important when you are responsible for every aspect of your own life. Laundry, grocery shopping, cooking, cleaning, and errands all cost energy. Spreading them across the week, using delivery services when available, and accepting that the apartment will not always be spotless are all reasonable adaptations, not signs of laziness.

Building a local support network takes time but pays for itself during the first bad flare. Identify at least one person near your home who knows your conditions and can help in an emergency: a neighbor, a friend, a coworker. Give them a copy of your emergency protocols. Let them know where your medications are stored. A phone call at 2 a.m. is a small ask when the alternative is calling 911 because no one nearby knows what is happening.

Paloma moved into her first apartment at age 22. She spent the first month terrified that something would go wrong and nobody would be there. Then she did something simple that changed everything. She baked cookies (from a safe recipe), brought them to her neighbor's door, introduced herself, and said, "I have a medical condition that sometimes causes emergencies. Would it be okay if I gave you my phone number in case I ever need help?" The neighbor said yes, learned the basics, and two months later was the person who drove Paloma to the ER during an anaphylaxis scare when the ambulance was 25 minutes away.

Independent does not mean alone. It means building the supports that let you stand on your own.

Summary

College with the trifecta requires early disability services registration, strategic dorm and meal plan accommodations, independent medication management, and the knowledge that medical leave is a legitimate strategy when health destabilizes.

Career planning should match the body you have, prioritizing flexibility, remote work potential, and low physical demand. Workplace accommodations under the ADA are available, and disclosure should happen on your terms and timeline.

Independent living requires systems for medical supply management, safe cooking, energy pacing, and a local support network that can respond during emergencies.

The goal of transition is not perfection. It is building a life with enough structure, support, and flexibility that the trifecta becomes something you manage rather than something that manages you. That life is possible. It takes planning, practice, and a willingness to ask for help when you need it.

You have spent this entire book learning how these conditions work, how to protect yourself at school, how to advocate with providers, and how to take care of your body and your mind. The skills you have built are the foundation. Now go build on it.

PART VI FOR THE PROFESSIONALS

Chapter 19 Recognize and Support Trifecta Students

The student in room 214 had been to the nurse's office nine times in October. Each visit followed the same pattern: she arrived pale and unsteady during second or third period, reported dizziness and nausea, rested for 20 minutes, drank some water, and returned to class. Her heart rate during these visits was consistently elevated, often above 120 beats per minute while sitting. She never had a fever. Her blood pressure was normal or low. No vomiting. No rash. No obvious infection.

The school nurse, a veteran of 16 years, documented each visit carefully. She noted the pattern. She mentioned it to the guidance counselor, who mentioned it to the assistant principal, who mentioned it to the girl's mother during a conference about her declining attendance. The mother, exhausted and confused, said she had taken her daughter to the pediatrician three times and been told everything was normal.

Nobody in the building connected the dots. The elevated heart rate upon standing. The pattern of morning worsening. The dizziness that resolved with rest and fluids. The normal lab work. The absence of fever or infection. These are the hallmarks of postural orthostatic tachycardia syndrome, and they were playing out in room 214 for months before anyone recognized them.

This chapter is written for you, the school nurse, the guidance counselor, the school psychologist, and the administrator who wants to support chronically ill students but may not have the clinical background to recognize what you are seeing. You are often the first professional to notice a pattern that the student's medical team has missed. Your observations can shorten a diagnostic process that otherwise takes years.

The trifecta of POTS, EDS, and MCAS presents in recognizable patterns in school settings. Once you know what to look for, you will start seeing it. And once you see it, you can change a student's life by asking the right questions and recommending the right referrals.

Learn the Patterns That Show Up at School

POTS in the school setting typically presents as a student who is fine while seated but becomes symptomatic upon standing. Watch for the student who gets dizzy in the hallway between classes, who needs to sit down during assemblies, who becomes pale and nauseated during morning periods, who reports headaches and fatigue that worsen as the day progresses (particularly on warm days or after physical activity), and whose heart rate, if you check it, is consistently 40 or more beats per minute higher standing than lying down. These students often show up in your office repeatedly with vague complaints that do not fit a clear pattern, until you recognize that the pattern is postural.

As we discussed in Chapter 1, POTS affects approximately one in every 100 teenagers, with onset most common between ages 12 and 15 and a strong female predominance (Boris & Bernadzikowski, 2018). It is far more common than most school health professionals realize. If you see a student with the profile described above, a simple screening test takes less than five minutes: measure the student's heart rate after lying quietly for five minutes, then measure it again after standing still for five and ten minutes. An increase of 40 or more beats per minute in an adolescent, combined with symptoms of dizziness, lightheadedness, or presyncope, strongly suggests POTS and warrants a referral to a pediatric cardiologist for formal evaluation.

EDS in the school setting shows up as the student who is unusually flexible ("double-jointed"), who sprains or dislocates joints without significant trauma, who bruises easily, who complains of joint pain that seems disproportionate to any visible injury, who has difficulty with handwriting due to finger and wrist instability, and who reports fatigue that does not correlate with sleep or activity level. Many of these students have been called clumsy, dramatic, or hypochondriac by adults who do not understand the condition. If a student reports frequent subluxations (partial dislocations) that they reduce themselves, that detail alone is strongly suggestive of a hypermobility disorder and merits referral to a geneticist or rheumatologist.

MCAS in the school setting is the hardest to recognize because its presentations are so varied. Watch for the student who has recurrent flushing, hives, or swelling that does not correspond to known allergens. Watch for unexplained GI distress (nausea, cramping, diarrhea) that fluctuates unpredictably. Watch for the student who reacts to environmental exposures that should be harmless: perfume, cleaning products, temperature changes, or physical exertion. If a student reports allergic-type reactions with negative allergy testing, MCAS should be considered. Referral to an allergist/immunologist with experience in mast cell disorders is appropriate.

The most telling pattern is when two or three of these presentations overlap in the same student. A student who is dizzy upon standing, has hypermobile joints, and develops hives after gym class is showing you the trifecta. That student needs a coordinated medical evaluation, not three separate dismissals.

One school nurse described the moment she started connecting the dots. "I had been seeing a girl for dizziness every Tuesday and Thursday, which were her PE days. I thought it was dehydration. Then I noticed she also came in with wrist pain that she said happened 'when I was just writing.' Then one day she came in covered in hives after running the mile. It was not until I talked to her mother that I learned she had already been diagnosed with POTS by a cardiologist, but nobody had evaluated the joints or the hives." The nurse referred the family to a geneticist and an allergist. Both diagnoses were confirmed within three months.

You do not need to diagnose these conditions. That is not your role. Your role is to recognize the pattern, document what you are seeing, communicate your observations to the family, and recommend that they pursue specific medical evaluations. A clear, specific referral recommendation from a school nurse carries weight with families and can accelerate a process that might otherwise stall for years.

Action Step: This week, review your visit log for the past three months. Identify any students who have visited your office five or more times with complaints of dizziness, fatigue, unexplained pain, or GI distress without a clear diagnosis. For each, check their heart rate lying down and standing. Note any patterns of morning worsening, postural symptoms, or environmental sensitivity. If the pattern fits, contact the family and recommend a specific referral.

Build Protocols Before You Need Them

Waiting until a trifecta student arrives in your building to develop protocols is like waiting until the fire to install the alarm. The protocols should be ready before the student walks through your door, because once they do, you will need them immediately.

Chapter 10 covered the nurse-family partnership in detail from the parent's perspective. This section addresses the same protocols from yours.

A POTS daily monitoring protocol should include a morning check-in (heart rate and blood pressure, lying and standing, with the student reporting their symptom severity on a 1 to 10 scale), documentation of each nurse visit during the day (time, presenting symptoms, vital signs, interventions provided, disposition), and criteria for sending the student home (sustained heart rate above a threshold set by the cardiologist, syncope or near-syncope that does not resolve with rest and fluids, or inability to maintain adequate hydration). Share the daily documentation with the family weekly and with the cardiologist monthly or as requested.

An EDS emergency response protocol should cover the three most common orthopedic events you will encounter. For finger or hand subluxations, the student can usually guide you through the reduction if they are experienced with it. Apply ice, provide a splint if needed, and document the event. For knee or ankle instability, immobilize the joint, apply ice, and contact the parent. Do not instruct the student to walk on an unstable joint. For shoulder subluxation or dislocation, apply a sling, provide ice, and contact the parent and physician. If the student cannot reduce the dislocation and is in significant pain, this may require emergency medical transport. In all cases, document what happened, what you did, and what the outcome was.

An MCAS emergency protocol should specify the location of the student's epinephrine auto-injectors (nurse's office and student's backpack, if authorized for self-carry), the criteria for administration as defined by the student's allergist, the steps after administration (call 911, position the student, notify parents, monitor for need for a second dose), and a clear note that mast cell activation episodes can look different from typical anaphylaxis. Flushing with severe GI distress and dizziness may not include the classic throat swelling and hives, but it can still be life-threatening.

Communication templates save time and improve consistency. Develop standard forms for daily vital sign logs, nurse visit documentation, teacher notification of accommodations, substitute teacher briefing sheets, field trip medical plans, and parent communication summaries. The templates in Appendix B of this book can be adapted for your building's specific needs.

Protect the Whole Student

Chronically ill students are at elevated risk for depression, anxiety, and social isolation. Research shows that adolescents with chronic medical conditions have two to three times the rate of depression and anxiety compared to their healthy peers (Pinquart & Shen, 2011). For trifecta students, the risk is compounded by the invisibility of their conditions, the unpredictability of their symptoms, and the social disruption caused by frequent absences.

As a school nurse or counselor, you are often the first person to notice the signs. Watch for withdrawal from friends and activities beyond what the medical condition explains. Watch for increasing reluctance to attend school on days when symptoms are actually manageable. Watch for statements that suggest hopelessness, self-blame, or loss of identity ("I used to be a good student," "Nobody understands," "What is the point").

The distinction between school avoidance driven by anxiety and school absence driven by illness matters and can be difficult to parse. A student with POTS who stays home because standing in the hallway makes them pass out is not avoiding school. They are avoiding syncope. A student with MCAS who refuses to enter the cafeteria because the smells make them vomit is not being difficult. They are protecting their body. Before labeling a chronically ill student's absences as "school refusal," consult with the family and the medical team to determine what role the illness is playing.

That said, some chronically ill students do develop genuine school-related anxiety that goes beyond symptom management. The experience of repeated public symptom episodes (fainting in the hallway, vomiting in class, leaving during a test) can create anticipatory dread that makes returning to school feel frightening even on good health days. When this pattern develops, it is a mental health concern that deserves support, not punishment. Connect the student with a school counselor or outside therapist who understands chronic illness, as discussed in Chapter 12. Frame the referral as support for the whole person, not as evidence that the illness is psychological.

Felix's school counselor made a point of checking in with him once a week, not about his grades or his absences, but about how he was doing. "She never tried to fix my POTS," Felix said later. "She just asked how I was handling it. That was enough." Sometimes the most powerful thing a school professional can do is ask a simple question and listen to the full answer.

Action Step: Identify one student in your building who has a chronic medical condition and who you have not checked in with personally in the past month. Schedule a brief, private conversation this week. Ask how they are doing, not medically but personally. Listen without solving. That conversation may be the first time anyone at school has asked.

Summary

The trifecta presents in recognizable school patterns: postural symptoms (POTS), joint instability with chronic pain (EDS), and unexplained allergic-type reactions (MCAS). When two or three patterns overlap in the same student, the trifecta should be considered and a coordinated medical referral recommended.

Protocols for daily monitoring, orthopedic emergencies, and mast cell activation emergencies should be developed before a trifecta student arrives, using templates that any staff member can follow.

Chronically ill students carry elevated risk for depression, anxiety, and social isolation. The line between illness-driven absence and anxiety-driven avoidance requires careful assessment with input from the family and medical team. School refusal labels should not be applied without this assessment.

Simple, regular check-ins from a trusted school professional can make a meaningful difference in a chronically ill student's emotional well-being. Ask how they are doing. Then listen.

Chapter 20 Screen Treat and Transition Together

Dr. Reyes had followed Zoe for three years. She was an excellent pediatric cardiologist who had diagnosed Zoe's POTS at age 13, stabilized her heart rate with a combination of fludrocortisone and midodrine, and worked with the school to develop an exercise protocol based on the modified CHOP program. By every cardiology measure, Zoe was doing well.

But Zoe was not doing well. She was still fatigued beyond what her POTS explained. She still had abdominal pain and nausea that the GI specialist attributed to "functional" causes. Her skin flushed unpredictably, and she had developed new food intolerances that appeared and disappeared without logic. Her joints ached, particularly her fingers and knees, but the rheumatologist had found no inflammation and discharged her.

At a routine follow-up, Zoe's mother said something that changed the conversation. "I have been reading about something called the trifecta. POTS with EDS and mast cell activation syndrome. Zoe has symptoms of all three. Has anyone screened her for the other two?"

Dr. Reyes paused. She had not. She had treated the POTS competently within her specialty, but she had not connected Zoe's remaining symptoms to conditions outside her primary focus. The flushing, the food intolerances, the GI distress pointed toward MCAS. The joint pain, the hypermobility she had noticed but not formally assessed, and the family history of "double-jointed" relatives pointed toward EDS.

Within four months, Zoe had all three diagnoses. Within six months, with treatment adjusted to address the full trifecta, her fatigue improved by half and her school attendance rose from 60% to 85%.

This chapter is written for pediatric healthcare teams: cardiologists, rheumatologists, allergists, geneticists, primary care physicians, nurse practitioners, and physician assistants who care for adolescents with any one of these conditions. The core message is simple. If you see one, screen for the others. The research supports it, the clinical outcomes reward it, and the families desperately need it.

Screen for the Full Picture

The evidence for co-occurrence is strong enough to justify routine screening. As we reviewed in Chapter 1, 31% of patients with both POTS and EDS also met criteria for MCAS in one study, compared to only 2% of patients without POTS or EDS (Cheung & Vadas, 2015). The association between hypermobile EDS and POTS is well-established, with estimates suggesting that 30% to 80% of hEDS patients also have some form of autonomic dysfunction (Roma et al., 2018). And while formal prevalence data for the full trifecta in pediatric populations remain limited, clinical experience at specialized centers suggests the clustering is common enough that screening should be standard practice.

If you are a cardiologist managing a teen with POTS, screen for EDS and MCAS. The EDS screen can be as simple as performing a Beighton score at a routine visit and asking about joint pain, dislocations, easy bruising, skin fragility, and family history of hypermobility. If the Beighton score is 5 or above in an adolescent and systemic features are present, refer to a geneticist or a rheumatologist experienced in hEDS evaluation. For MCAS screening, ask about flushing, hives, unexplained GI distress, food intolerances, and reactions to environmental exposures (heat, fragrances, exercise). If the symptom pattern is suggestive, refer to an allergist/immunologist and consider ordering baseline tryptase and, during a flare, a 24-hour urine collection for histamine metabolites and prostaglandin D2 metabolites.

If you are a geneticist or rheumatologist managing a teen with EDS, screen for POTS and MCAS. POTS screening requires only a set of vital signs: measure heart rate lying down after five minutes of rest, then standing at one, three, five, and ten minutes. An increase of 40 or more beats per minute in an adolescent with symptoms of orthostatic intolerance warrants cardiology referral. MCAS screening follows the same approach described above.

If you are an allergist managing a teen with MCAS, screen for POTS and EDS. Many MCAS patients describe orthostatic intolerance that is attributed to mast cell-mediated vasodilation but may reflect concurrent POTS. The Beighton score and a brief musculoskeletal history can identify hypermobility that merits further evaluation.

The screening adds minutes to a visit. The results can save years.

Action Step: At your next clinical team meeting, propose adding a standardized trifecta screening question set to the intake form for any adolescent presenting with POTS, EDS, or MCAS. Three to five additional questions per condition can flag the need for cross-specialty referral without adding significant time to the visit.

Coordinate Care Across Specialties

The trifecta does not fit neatly into any single medical specialty. Cardiology manages the POTS. Genetics or rheumatology manages the EDS. Allergy/immunology manages the MCAS. Primary care manages the whole patient. Physical therapy manages the rehabilitation. And nobody, in many cases, is managing the interactions among these conditions and their treatments.

The "medical home" model, in which a primary care provider serves as the central coordinator for all specialist care, is the recommended framework for adolescents with complex chronic conditions (American Academy of Pediatrics, 2002). For trifecta teens, the medical home means one provider who receives all specialist notes, reviews the complete medication list for cross-condition interactions (the treatment conflicts discussed in Chapter 7), monitors school functioning and mental health alongside physical symptoms, and initiates referrals when new symptoms suggest involvement of an additional condition.

Multidisciplinary clinic models, where multiple specialists see the patient on the same day in the same location, offer the most efficient care for complex patients. A few centers now offer combined dysautonomia-connective tissue-mast cell clinics where a cardiologist, geneticist, and immunologist evaluate the patient sequentially and then confer on a unified treatment plan. These clinics are rare, but they are growing. If your institution does not have one, consider whether the patient volume justifies creating a monthly combined clinic or a virtual case conference where specialists review shared patients together.

Telehealth integration can extend the reach of specialized trifecta care. A primary care provider in a rural community can manage day-to-day care while a trifecta-experienced specialist at a distant center provides quarterly telehealth consultations, reviews data remotely, and adjusts the treatment plan. This hybrid model, described in detail in Chapter 16, depends on clear communication channels between the local and remote providers, shared access to medical records, and defined roles for who manages what.

Hugo's care team included a pediatric cardiologist, a geneticist, an allergist, a physical therapist, a school nurse, and his pediatrician. For two years, each provider worked independently. When his pediatrician agreed to serve as coordinator and began receiving copies of all specialist notes, the team discovered that Hugo's allergist had increased his antihistamine dose at the same visit where his cardiologist had started a new beta-blocker. The combination was causing excessive sedation that neither specialist had attributed to their own intervention because neither knew about the other's change. A five-minute phone call between the three providers resolved the issue. Coordination costs less time than confusion.

Plan the Transition From the Beginning

The transition from pediatric to adult care should not begin at the patient's 18th birthday. It should begin the day of diagnosis.

From the first appointment, frame the patient's care in the context of a future where they will manage their conditions independently. Use age-appropriate language to explain diagnoses to the teen directly, not only to the parent. As the patient matures, gradually shift the conversation so that the teen is the primary participant and the parent is the observer, as we described in Chapter 15 with Elio's cardiologist.

Standardized transition readiness assessments can help you track progress. Tools such as the TRAQ (Transition Readiness Assessment Questionnaire) or the STARx (Self-Management and Transition to Adulthood with Treatment) measure a young patient's knowledge of their conditions, their ability to manage medications, their comfort communicating with providers independently, and their understanding of insurance and healthcare systems (Sawicki et al., 2011; Cohen et al., 2015). Administering these annually starting at age 14 identifies gaps early enough to address them before the transition.

The warm handoff is the single most effective strategy for preventing the care gap that occurs during transfer to adult providers. Rather than giving the family a list of adult provider names and wishing them well, schedule a joint appointment or a phone consultation where you introduce the patient's case directly to the receiving adult provider. Share the medication history, the treatment successes and failures, the baseline symptom levels, and the specific concerns that the family and patient have about the transition. This conversation gives the adult provider a running start and gives the patient confidence that they are not starting over from zero.

Oscar's transition, described in Chapter 16, went poorly because no warm handoff occurred. Eloise's transition, from the same chapter, went well because her pediatric cardiologist called the adult electrophysiologist before the first visit. The difference was one phone call. It cost 15 minutes. It saved months of disruption.

Post-transfer follow-up closes the final gap. After the patient has been seen by the adult provider, check in with the family by phone or patient portal message. Ask how the first appointment went. Ask if the adult provider had questions that you can answer. Some pediatric practices maintain a six-month open-door policy where they will see the patient for acute issues if the adult provider is not yet fully up to speed. This safety net reduces the risk of the patient falling through the cracks during the most vulnerable period of the transition.

Action Step: For every adolescent patient in your practice with POTS, EDS, or MCAS, document their current transition readiness score and the date of their next scheduled transition assessment. If no assessment has been done and the patient is 14 or older, schedule one within the next two visits. If the patient is 17 or older and no adult provider has been identified, begin the referral process now.

Summary

If you see one condition in the trifecta, screen for the other two. The co-occurrence rates are high enough to justify routine cross-condition screening at every adolescent visit for POTS, EDS, or MCAS.

Coordinated care across specialties prevents the treatment conflicts, medication interactions, and communication gaps that harm trifecta patients when each specialist works in isolation. The medical home model, multidisciplinary clinics, and telehealth integration all offer structures for this coordination.

Transition planning should begin at diagnosis, not at age 18. Standardized readiness assessments, gradual transfer of responsibility to the teen, warm handoffs to adult providers, and post-transfer follow-up are evidence-based practices that reduce the care gap.

The families sitting across from you have often spent years fighting for a diagnosis. They have educated themselves, researched treatments, and advocated through systems that were not designed for their child's conditions. They are tired. They are resourceful. And they are counting on you to see the full picture. Do not let the limits of your specialty become the limits of your patient's care.

APPENDICES

Appendix A Condition Specific Accommodations Checklists

POTS School Accommodations Checklist

Attendance: Modified attendance policy distinguishing medically documented absences from unexcused absences. Flexible scheduling with late start option. Reduced course load during unstable periods. Homebound instruction protocol for extended flares. Virtual or hybrid attendance options when available.

Hydration and Nutrition: Water bottle permitted on desk in all classes at all times. Electrolyte drinks permitted in classrooms. Salty snacks permitted during class. Electrolyte refill access without restriction. Cafeteria accommodations for high-sodium meal options.

Physical Environment: Elevator key or code for all multi-story buildings. Classroom seating near the door for easy exit. Locker on the ground floor near primary classrooms. Permission to stand, walk, or change position during class. Temperature-controlled testing and classroom environments. Proximity to the nurse's office considered in scheduling.

Academic: Extended time on tests and assignments (recommended: 50% additional). Testing in a quiet, cool room with water, electrolyte drinks, and snack access. Permission to stand or walk during tests. Note-taking accommodations (peer notes, recorded lectures, laptop use). Modified assignment deadlines during documented flare periods. Alternative assessment methods when brain fog is severe.

Physical Education: Modified PE program with physician-prescribed exercise plan. Recumbent exercise alternatives (cycling, swimming, rowing). Heart rate monitoring during activity with a defined stopping threshold. Cool gymnasium or outdoor environment for PE. Option for alternative PE credit through documented home exercise logs.

Emergency: Syncope response protocol posted in nurse's office and shared with all teachers. Permission to lie down with elevated legs immediately upon symptom onset. Access to electrolytes, water, and blood pressure monitoring in the nurse's office. Parent notification protocol for syncope events.

EDS School Accommodations Checklist

Physical Environment: Ergonomic seating (supportive chair, ability to alternate sitting and standing). Locker placement at accessible height near primary classrooms. Duplicate textbook sets (one at school, one at home). Rolling backpack or permission to use a cart. Avoidance of carrying heavy materials between classes. Elevator access for all multi-story buildings.

Academic: Laptop use for all written work (keyboarding instead of handwriting). Extended time on handwritten assignments if laptop is not available. Note-taking accommodations (peer notes, recorded lectures). Scribe for extended writing tasks during flare periods. Permission to use voice-to-text software.

Physical Education: Modified PE with physician-prescribed activity plan. Prohibition of contact sports and high-impact activities. Joint protection modifications for all physical activities. Bracing and taping permitted during activity. Immediate access to ice packs and elastic wraps. Adaptive PE credit through swimming, recumbent cycling, or yoga with modifications.

Safety: Joint subluxation and dislocation response protocol posted in nurse's office. First aid supplies (ice packs, elastic wraps, splints) accessible in nurse's office and gymnasium. Staff training on EDS first response (do not instruct student to "walk it off" or "stretch it out"). Avoidance of activities requiring repetitive joint stress (rope climbing, heavy lifting, sustained gripping). Backpack weight not to exceed 10% to 15% of body weight.

Pain Management: Access to prescribed pain medication during school hours. Permission to use ice packs and heating pads in the classroom. Scheduled rest breaks during the school day. Nurse visit protocol for pain flare management.

MCAS School Accommodations Checklist

Environmental: Fragrance-reduced classroom and immediate seating area. Advance notice of cleaning chemical use in the student's building area. Avoidance of exposure to known chemical triggers in science labs and art rooms. Temperature-controlled classrooms (avoiding both extreme heat and cold). Air filtration or open windows in the student's primary classrooms when possible.

Food and Medication: Permission to bring home-prepared meals and snacks. Cafeteria communication regarding ingredients and food allergens. Access to a safe eating space if the cafeteria environment is triggering. Water and electrolyte drinks permitted in all classes. Self-carry authorization for antihistamines (H1 and H2) and epinephrine auto-injectors. Nurse-administered medications on schedule as prescribed. Medical refrigerator access for temperature-sensitive medications.

Emergency: MCAS flare and anaphylaxis response protocol posted in nurse's office and shared with all teachers. Epinephrine auto-injectors stored in nurse's office and in student's backpack (if authorized). Criteria for epinephrine administration clearly defined by the student's allergist. Post-administration steps: call 911, position student, notify parents, monitor for second dose. Staff training on recognizing atypical mast cell activation (flushing with GI distress, progressive hives without respiratory symptoms, rapid-onset fatigue with dizziness).

Academic: Extended time on tests and assignments during flare periods. Modified assignment deadlines during documented flares. Testing in a fragrance-reduced, temperature-controlled room.

Permission to leave class immediately during onset of symptoms without requesting permission.

Combined Trifecta Accommodations Master Checklist

All items from the POTS, EDS, and MCAS checklists above, plus the following coordination items:

Care coordination: Designated 504 coordinator who understands all three conditions. Single Individualized Health Plan (IHP) that addresses all three conditions in one document. Single Emergency Care Plan (ECP) that covers syncope, dislocation, and anaphylaxis. Annual review meeting with school nurse, 504 coordinator, parents, and at least one treating specialist (by phone if in-person is not possible).

Communication: One-page trifecta condition summary on file in the main office, nurse's office, and with all of the student's teachers. Substitute teacher briefing protocol that covers all three conditions. Field trip medical plan for each off-campus event. Parent-nurse communication schedule (weekly email or as needed during flares).

Medication coordination: Complete medication list posted in the nurse's office, including medication interactions across conditions. Timing schedule for all medications administered during school hours. Clear documentation of which medications the student self-carries and which are nurse-administered.

Appendix B Templates and Forms

Model 504 Plan for Trifecta Teens

Student Name: _______________

Date of Birth: _______________

School: _______________

Grade: _______________

Date of Plan: _______________

Review Date: _______________

Medical Diagnoses: Postural Orthostatic Tachycardia Syndrome (POTS), Ehlers-Danlos Syndrome (hypermobile type/HSD), Mast Cell Activation Syndrome (MCAS)

Treating Providers: (list names, specialties, and contact information for each)

Statement of Disability: The student named above has been diagnosed with three chronic medical conditions that substantially limit multiple major life activities including standing, walking, concentrating, learning, eating, breathing, and the operation of cardiovascular, immune, neurological, and musculoskeletal bodily functions.

Accommodations Provided: (select and customize from the checklists in Appendix A based on the individual student's needs)

Attendance accommodations: _______________

Physical environment accommodations: _______________

Academic accommodations: _______________

Physical education accommodations: _______________

Food and hydration accommodations: _______________

Medication accommodations: _______________

Emergency protocol: (see attached Emergency Care Plan)

Signatures:

Parent/Guardian: _______________ Date: _______________

504 Coordinator: _______________ Date: _______________

School Nurse: _______________ Date: _______________

Principal/Designee: _______________ Date: _______________

Model IEP Goals for Trifecta Students

Self-Advocacy Goal: By (date), the student will independently communicate their accommodation needs to at least three teachers per semester, as documented by teacher confirmation and student self-report.

Health Management Goal: By (date), the student will independently monitor and record their daily vital signs (heart rate, symptom severity) with 80% accuracy over a four-week period, as measured by the school nurse's review of the student's health log.

Academic Independence Goal: By (date), the student will complete 90% of modified assignments during flare periods within the extended deadline, as documented by teacher grade records.

Transition Readiness Goal: By (date), the student will demonstrate the ability to explain their three medical conditions, list their current medications, and describe their emergency protocol to a new provider, as assessed by a role-play evaluation with the school nurse or counselor.

Model Individualized Health Plan (IHP)

Student Name: _______________

Date of Birth: _______________

Grade: _______________

Date of Plan: _______________

Prepared by: (School Nurse Name, RN)

Diagnoses:

1. Postural Orthostatic Tachycardia Syndrome (POTS): Diagnosed (date) by (provider). Characterized by heart rate increase of _____ bpm upon standing, chronic dizziness, fatigue, brain fog, and presyncope.

2. Ehlers-Danlos Syndrome (type): Diagnosed (date) by (provider). Characterized by joint hypermobility, chronic pain, frequent subluxations of (joints), easy bruising, and fatigue.

3. Mast Cell Activation Syndrome: Diagnosed (date) by (provider). Characterized by recurrent flushing, hives, GI distress, and reactions to (known triggers). History of anaphylaxis: Yes / No.

Current Medications Administered at School:

Medication, Dose, Time, Route, Stored in: (list each)

Daily Monitoring Protocol: Morning check-in with nurse. Heart rate lying and standing. Symptom severity scale (1 to 10). Documentation in daily log. Notify teachers if baseline is poor.

Triggers to Avoid: (list student-specific triggers: heat, fragrances, specific foods, exercise intensity, etc.)

Activity Restrictions: (list physician-specified restrictions for PE, recess, field trips)

When to Contact Parent: (list specific criteria)

When to Call 911: (list specific criteria: syncope with injury, sustained heart rate above _____, signs of anaphylaxis, dislocation that cannot be reduced)

Model Emergency Care Plan (ECP)

Student Name and Photo: _______________

Grade and Classroom: _______________

Date: _______________

Diagnoses: POTS, EDS (type), MCAS

Emergency Contacts: (parent names, phone numbers, backup contacts)

Physicians: (primary care, cardiologist, allergist, with phone numbers)

Emergency 1: Syncope (Fainting)

Do: Lower student to the floor. Elevate legs above heart level. Loosen tight clothing. Offer water and electrolytes when alert. Monitor heart rate. Stay with the student.

Do Not: Attempt to keep the student upright. Restrict the student from lying down. Leave the student unattended.

Call 911 if: Student does not regain consciousness within 2 minutes. Student is injured from the fall. Heart rate remains above _____ bpm for more than 15 minutes after lying down.

Call Parent: After every syncope event.

Emergency 2: Joint Dislocation or Subluxation

Do: Help the student to a comfortable position. Apply ice. Immobilize the joint with a splint or sling if available. Allow the student to self-reduce if they are experienced. Document the event.

Do Not: Force the joint back into place. Instruct the student to move the affected limb. Tell the student to "walk it off."

Call 911 if: The student is in severe pain and cannot reduce the dislocation. There is visible deformity or loss of circulation (numbness, color change in fingers or toes).

Call Parent: After every dislocation. After subluxations if the student is in significant pain or unable to return to class.

Emergency 3: Mast Cell Activation / Anaphylaxis

Do: Administer epinephrine auto-injector if the student has two or more of the following: progressive hives or flushing, GI distress (cramping, vomiting, diarrhea), throat tightness or difficulty breathing, dizziness with blood pressure drop, rapid heart rate. Call 911 immediately after administering epinephrine. Position the student lying flat with legs elevated (unless breathing is compromised, in which case allow the student to sit up). Notify parents. Monitor for need for a second epinephrine dose (available after 5 to 15 minutes if symptoms do not improve). Stay with the student until emergency medical services arrive.

Do Not: Wait to see if symptoms improve before administering epinephrine. Administer antihistamines as a substitute for epinephrine during a severe reaction. Leave the student unattended. Allow the student to stand or walk.

Epinephrine Location: Nurse's office (drawer/cabinet) and student's backpack (if authorized).

Physician Letter Template for School Accommodations

(Provider Letterhead)

Date: _______________

To Whom It May Concern:

I am writing to support the request for school accommodations for (Student Name), date of birth (DOB), who is a patient in my practice.

(Student Name) has been diagnosed with the following conditions: (list diagnoses with dates of diagnosis).

These conditions substantially limit the following major life activities: (list affected activities with brief explanation of how each condition contributes).

Based on my clinical assessment, I recommend the following accommodations to allow (Student Name) to access their education safely and effectively: (list specific recommended accommodations, organized by category).

I am available to discuss these recommendations with the school team and to provide additional documentation if needed. Please contact my office at (phone number) with any questions.

Sincerely,

(Provider Name, Credentials)

(Practice Name)

(Phone and Fax)

Medical Summary Template for Transition

(See Chapter 15 for instructions on completing this document)

Full Legal Name: _______________

Date of Birth: _______________

Emergency Contact: _______________

Insurance Information: _______________

Diagnoses (with dates of diagnosis):

1. _______________
2. _______________
3. _______________

Current Medications:

Medication, Dose, Frequency, Purpose, Prescribing Provider: (list each)

Known Allergies and Adverse Drug Reactions: _______________

Current Specialists:

Provider Name, Specialty, Phone, Last Seen: (list each)

Emergency Protocols:

For syncope: _______________

For dislocation: _______________

For anaphylaxis: _______________

Surgical History: _______________

Most Recent Lab Results (with dates): _______________

Current 504/IEP Status: _______________

Primary Care Provider: _______________

Date Last Updated: _______________

Appendix C Medication Quick Reference

POTS Medications

Fludrocortisone (Florinef): Synthetic mineralocorticoid. Expands blood volume through sodium and water retention. Typical adolescent starting dose: 0.1 mg daily. Monitor potassium levels. Common side effects: headache, swelling, low potassium. School-day note: best taken in the morning; does not typically cause classroom-relevant side effects.

Midodrine (ProAmatine): Alpha-1 agonist vasoconstrictor. Reduces blood pooling by tightening blood vessels. Typical adolescent dose: 2.5 to 10 mg, two to three times daily. Common side effects: scalp tingling, goosebumps, urinary urgency. School-day note: takes effect within one hour, lasts approximately four hours. Timing around the school day is critical. Should not be taken before lying down (raises supine blood pressure).

Metoprolol and Propranolol (Beta-blockers): Reduce heart rate. May help hyperadrenergic POTS. Common side effects: fatigue, exercise intolerance, cognitive dulling, cold extremities. School-day note: cognitive side effects can impair concentration and test performance. Discuss timing with prescriber to minimize school-hour impact.

Ivabradine (Corlanor): Selective sinus node inhibitor. Reduces heart rate without lowering blood pressure or causing the cognitive effects of beta-blockers. Typical adolescent dose: 2.5 to 7.5 mg twice daily. Common side effects: visual disturbances (luminous phenomena), bradycardia. School-day note: generally well tolerated in the classroom; visual side effects are usually mild and transient.

Pyridostigmine (Mestinon): Acetylcholinesterase inhibitor. Improves blood vessel constriction and reduces heart rate upon standing. Typical adolescent dose: 30 to 60 mg, two to three times daily. Common side effects: GI cramping, diarrhea, increased salivation. School-day note: GI side effects may increase bathroom visit frequency.

MCAS Medications

H1 Antihistamines (cetirizine, fexofenadine, loratadine): Block histamine at H1 receptors. Reduce itching, flushing, hives, nasal congestion. Second-generation agents (cetirizine, fexofenadine, loratadine) are preferred for daytime use because they are less sedating. School-day note: cetirizine can cause mild drowsiness in some patients. If drowsiness occurs, fexofenadine is typically the least sedating alternative.

H2 Antihistamines (famotidine): Block histamine at H2 receptors in the GI tract. Reduce nausea, acid reflux, and GI cramping. Typical dose: 20 to 40 mg, once or twice daily. School-day note: no significant classroom-relevant side effects.

Cromolyn Sodium (Gastrocrom): Mast cell stabilizer taken orally before meals. Prevents mast cell degranulation in the GI tract. Typical dose: 100 to 200 mg, 15 to 30 minutes before meals. School-day note: must be taken before lunch at school. Requires planning and possibly nurse administration.

Ketotifen: Antihistamine with mast cell stabilizing properties. Typical dose: 1 to 2 mg, once or twice daily. Common side effects: drowsiness (often improves after two to four weeks), weight gain. School-day note: drowsiness is common initially. If used, evening dosing may be preferred until tolerance develops.

Montelukast (Singulair): Leukotriene receptor antagonist. Reduces respiratory and nasal symptoms. Typical dose: 10 mg daily. Common side effects: headache; rare reports of behavioral changes and mood disturbance (FDA boxed warning). School-day note: monitor for mood changes; taken once daily, usually in the evening.

Epinephrine Auto-Injector (EpiPen, Auvi-Q): Rescue medication for anaphylaxis or severe mast cell activation. Dose: 0.3 mg (standard) or 0.15 mg (junior). Should be carried at all times by students at risk for severe reactions. School-day note: stored in nurse's office and student's backpack (if authorized). All staff in contact with the student should know its location and administration steps.

EDS Pain Management Options

Topical lidocaine patches (Lidoderm): Applied directly to painful joints. Provides localized pain relief without systemic effects. No significant classroom-relevant side effects.

Topical anti-inflammatory gels (diclofenac gel): Applied to painful joints. Note: NSAIDs (oral or topical) should be used with caution in MCAS patients, as some patients react to NSAIDs.

Low-dose naltrexone (LDN): Off-label use for chronic pain and neuroinflammation. Typical dose: 1 to 4.5 mg at bedtime. May take four to eight weeks for full effect. Generally well tolerated. School-day note: taken at bedtime; no classroom-relevant side effects.

Acetaminophen (Tylenol): Over-the-counter pain relief. Generally safe for trifecta patients. Avoid exceeding 2,000 mg per day in adolescents. School-day note: may be nurse-administered with physician authorization.

Cross-Condition Drug Interactions to Monitor

Beta-blockers combined with sedating antihistamines: Additive fatigue and cognitive dulling. Monitor school performance closely.

Fludrocortisone combined with cromolyn sodium: No direct interaction, but fludrocortisone-induced fluid retention may worsen MCAS-related GI bloating. Monitor GI symptoms.

Midodrine combined with epinephrine: Both raise blood pressure. After epinephrine administration during anaphylaxis, monitor blood pressure closely if the patient is also taking midodrine.

NSAIDs (ibuprofen, naproxen) in MCAS patients: Can trigger mast cell activation in some patients. Use acetaminophen as the first-line over-the-counter pain reliever unless the allergist has confirmed NSAID tolerance.

Appendix D Resources

National Organizations and Foundations

Dysautonomia International: Information, research funding, and support for dysautonomia conditions including POTS. Provider directory. School accommodations resources. www.dysautonomiainternational.org

The Ehlers-Danlos Society: Global organization providing information, support, and research advocacy for all types of EDS and HSD. Provider directory. www.ehlers-danlos.com

The Mast Cell Disease Society (TMS): Education, research funding, and support for all mast cell diseases including MCAS. Provider directory. www.tmsforacure.org

Standing Up to POTS: Patient advocacy organization with school accommodation guides, research updates, and community support. www.standinguptopots.org

Mast Cell Action: UK-based organization with MCAS information, trigger management resources, and support. www.mastcellaction.org

Online Support Communities for Teens and Parents

Dysautonomia International Support Groups: Facebook-based groups for parents, teens, and adults with POTS and related conditions. Age-specific groups available.

The Ehlers-Danlos Society Community: Online forums and social media communities connecting EDS patients and families worldwide.

POTS subreddit (r/POTS): Reddit community with peer support, questions, and shared experiences. Monitor teen engagement and verify medical claims through professional sources.

Mast Cell Disease Society online community: Forum-based support for MCAS patients and caregivers.

Provider Directories and Finding Specialists

Dysautonomia International Provider Directory: Searchable database of providers who treat POTS and related dysautonomias.

The EDS Clinic: Multi-state clinic specializing in the trifecta. Telehealth and in-person options. www.eds.clinic

EDS-Aware Provider List (The Ehlers-Danlos Society): Global directory of providers with EDS experience.

The Mast Cell Disease Society Provider List: Directory of allergists and immunologists with mast cell disease experience.

Disability Scholarship Databases

Disability Scholarships (disabilityscholarships.us): Searchable database of scholarships for students with disabilities.

The Ehlers-Danlos Society Scholarship Program: Annual scholarships for students with EDS.

Dysautonomia International Kevin J. Klos Memorial Scholarship: Annual scholarship for students with dysautonomia.

HEATH Resource Center at the National Youth Transitions Center: Information on postsecondary education for students with disabilities.

Adaptive Sports Programs

Adaptive Sports USA: National organization promoting adaptive sports and recreation for people with physical disabilities.

Move United: Nationwide network of adaptive sports programs including swimming, cycling, and fitness.

Local YMCA/YWCA: Many locations offer adaptive fitness programs and inclusive swimming.

Recommended Reading

For Teens: "The Chronic Illness Workbook for Teens" by Rachel Zoffness, PhD. Practical strategies for managing the emotional and social impact of chronic illness.

For Parents: "Palliative Care for Chronic Illness" series. Medical management guides for specific conditions.

For Professionals: Boris, J. R., & Moak, J. P. (2022). "Pediatric Postural Orthostatic Tachycardia Syndrome: Where We Stand." Pediatrics. A clinical review of current evidence for pediatric POTS management.

For All Readers: Malfait, F., et al. (2017). "The 2017 International Classification of the Ehlers-Danlos Syndromes." The definitive classification paper for EDS types and diagnostic criteria.

Appendix E Glossary of Medical Terms

Anaphylaxis: A severe, potentially life-threatening allergic reaction that can affect multiple body systems simultaneously. Symptoms may include throat swelling, difficulty breathing, rapid heart rate, low blood pressure, hives, and GI distress. Requires immediate treatment with epinephrine.

Autonomic Nervous System (ANS): The part of the nervous system that controls body functions you do not think about: heart rate, blood pressure, digestion, temperature regulation, and blood vessel constriction. Dysautonomia means this system is not working properly.

Beighton Score: A clinical tool used to measure joint hypermobility. It tests flexibility at nine points on the body (fifth fingers, thumbs, elbows, knees, and spine). A score of 5 or more out of 9 in adolescents suggests generalized hypermobility.

Brain Fog: A common term for the cognitive impairment experienced by many POTS patients. Includes difficulty concentrating, slow processing speed, trouble finding words, and reduced working memory. Caused by reduced blood flow to the brain.

Connective Tissue: The biological material that gives structure and support to joints, skin, blood vessels, and internal organs. Made primarily of collagen. In EDS, connective tissue is too stretchy or fragile.

Deconditioning: The loss of cardiovascular and muscular fitness that occurs when physical activity is reduced, often due to illness. Deconditioning worsens POTS symptoms. Reconditioning through graduated exercise is a primary treatment.

Dislocation: When a joint comes completely out of its normal position. Requires repositioning (reduction). Common in EDS, especially in shoulders, kneecaps, and fingers.

Dysautonomia: A general term for conditions in which the autonomic nervous system does not function properly. POTS is one form of dysautonomia.

Ehlers-Danlos Syndrome (EDS): A group of 13 inherited connective tissue disorders characterized by joint hypermobility, skin fragility, and tissue weakness. The hypermobile type (hEDS) is most commonly associated with the trifecta.

Epinephrine: A hormone and medication (also called adrenaline) that reverses the symptoms of anaphylaxis by constricting blood vessels, opening airways, and increasing heart rate. Delivered via auto-injector (EpiPen, Auvi-Q).

Flare: A period of worsened symptoms. Flares can last hours, days, or weeks. They may be triggered by identifiable causes or may occur without clear provocation.

Fludrocortisone: A synthetic mineralocorticoid medication that increases blood volume by promoting sodium and water retention. Used in POTS management.

Gastroparesis: Delayed emptying of the stomach, causing nausea, bloating, and early fullness. Can occur in EDS and POTS due to autonomic dysfunction affecting gut motility.

Histamine: A chemical released by mast cells during immune activation. Causes itching, flushing, swelling, increased stomach acid, and blood vessel dilation. Overproduction of histamine is a hallmark of MCAS.

Hypermobility: Joints that bend beyond the normal range of motion. Often called "double-jointed." When accompanied by symptoms (pain, dislocations, fatigue), it may indicate EDS or hypermobility spectrum disorder.

Hypermobility Spectrum Disorder (HSD): A condition characterized by symptomatic joint hypermobility that does not meet the full diagnostic criteria for hEDS. Managed similarly to hEDS.

Interoception: The ability to perceive and interpret internal body signals such as hunger, thirst, pain, temperature, and heart rate. Often atypical in neurodivergent individuals.

Mast Cell: A type of immune cell found in tissues throughout the body. Mast cells store and release chemical mediators (including histamine) in response to perceived threats. In MCAS, mast cells release mediators inappropriately.

Mast Cell Activation Syndrome (MCAS): A condition in which mast cells become overactive and release chemical mediators too easily, causing symptoms across multiple body systems. Diagnosed based on clinical symptoms, elevated mast cell mediator levels, and response to mast cell targeted medications.

Midodrine: A vasoconstrictor medication that tightens blood vessels and reduces blood pooling. Used in POTS management to reduce orthostatic symptoms.

Orthostatic Intolerance (OI): Symptoms that occur upon standing, including dizziness, lightheadedness, palpitations, nausea, and visual changes. A core feature of POTS.

POTS (Postural Orthostatic Tachycardia Syndrome): A form of dysautonomia characterized by an excessive increase in heart rate upon standing (40 or more bpm in adolescents) without significant blood pressure drop, along with symptoms of orthostatic intolerance lasting at least three months.

Presyncope: The feeling of nearly fainting. Symptoms include dizziness, tunnel vision, warmth, nausea, and sweating. In POTS, presyncope is common and may or may not progress to actual fainting.

Proprioception: The body's sense of where its parts are in space. Important for joint stability. Often impaired in EDS, contributing to clumsiness and increased injury risk.

Subluxation: A partial dislocation in which a joint slides partially out of position and then returns. Common in EDS. Can be painful and may cause temporary loss of function.

Syncope: Fainting. A temporary loss of consciousness caused by reduced blood flow to the brain. In POTS, syncope can occur upon standing, during prolonged standing, or in warm environments.

Tilt Table Test: A diagnostic test for POTS in which the patient lies flat on a table that is then tilted to a near-upright position while heart rate and blood pressure are monitored. Used to measure the heart rate response to standing.

Trifecta: The common co-occurrence of POTS, EDS, and MCAS in the same patient. Also called the triad. These three conditions frequently cluster together and create interconnected symptom patterns.

Tryptase: An enzyme released by mast cells. Measured in blood tests as a marker of mast cell activation. Elevated levels during symptomatic episodes support a diagnosis of MCAS, though many MCAS patients have normal baseline tryptase levels.

504 Plan: A plan developed under Section 504 of the Rehabilitation Act of 1973 that provides accommodations for students with disabilities in public schools. Designed to ensure equal access to education.

IEP (Individualized Education Program): A plan developed under the Individuals with Disabilities Education Act (IDEA) that provides specialized instruction and related services for students with disabilities who need more than accommodations alone.

IHP (Individualized Health Plan): A plan developed by the school nurse that outlines the day-to-day medical management a student needs during school hours, including medication schedules, monitoring protocols, and activity restrictions.

ECP (Emergency Care Plan): A plan that provides step-by-step instructions for responding to medical emergencies at school. For trifecta students, this typically covers syncope, joint dislocation, and anaphylaxis.

About the Author

James Philip McGowan is a researcher and writer focused on chronic illness education, adolescent health, and family advocacy. His work centers on translating clinical research into practical guidance that families, educators, and healthcare professionals can use in daily life. He holds a particular interest in conditions that are frequently underdiagnosed in young people, and he is committed to producing resources that close the gap between what medical science knows and what families can access.

References

- ACT, Inc. (n.d.). *Requesting accommodations for the ACT test.*
- ADA Amendments Act of 2008, Pub. L. No. 110-325, 122 Stat. 3553 (2008).
- American Academy of Pediatrics. (2002). The medical home. *Pediatrics, 110*(1 Pt 1), 184–186.
- American Academy of Pediatrics, American Academy of Family Physicians, & American College of Physicians. (2018). Supporting the health care transition from adolescence to adulthood in the medical home. *Pediatrics, 142*(5), e20182587.
- Benarroch, E. E. (2012). Postural tachycardia syndrome: A heterogeneous and multifactorial disorder. *Mayo Clinic Proceedings, 87*(12), 1214–1225.
- Boris, J. R., & Bernadzikowski, T. (2018). Demographics of a large pediatric postural orthostatic tachycardia syndrome program. *Cardiology in the Young, 28*(5), 668–674.
- Boris, J. R., & Moak, J. P. (2022). Pediatric postural orthostatic tachycardia syndrome: Where we stand. *Pediatrics, 150*(1), e2021054945.
- Casanova, E. L., Baeza-Velasco, C., Buchanan, C. B., & Casanova, M. F. (2020). The relationship between autism and Ehlers-Danlos syndromes/hypermobility spectrum disorders. *Journal of Personalized Medicine, 10*(4), 260.
- Castells, M., Giannetti, M. P., Hamilton, M. J., Novak, P., Pozdnyakova, O., Nicoloro-SantaBarbara, J., Jennings, S. V., Francomano, C., Kim, B., Glover, S. C., Galli, S. J., Maitland, A., White, A., Abonia, J. P., Slee, V., Valent, P., Butterfield, J. H., Carter, M., Metcalfe, D. D., Akin, C., Lyons, J. J., Togias, A., Wheatley, L., & Milner, J. D. (2024). Mast cell activation syndrome: Current understanding and research needs. *The Journal of Allergy and Clinical Immunology, 154*(2), 255–263.

- Castori, M., Morlino, S., Celletti, C., Celli, M., Morrone, A., Colombi, M., Dordoni, C., Sperduti, I., Ritelli, M., Venturini, M., Camerota, F., Celletti, F., & Grammatico, P. (2012). Management of pain and fatigue in the joint hypermobility syndrome (a.k.a. Ehlers-Danlos syndrome, hypermobility type): Principles and proposal for a multidisciplinary approach. *American Journal of Medical Genetics Part A, 158A*(8), 2055–2070.
- Cederlöf, M., Larsson, H., Lichtenstein, P., Almqvist, C., Serlachius, E., & Ludvigsson, J. F. (2016). Nationwide population-based cohort study of psychiatric disorders in individuals with Ehlers-Danlos syndrome or hypermobility syndrome and their siblings. *BMC Psychiatry, 16*, 207.
- Cheung, I., & Vadas, P. (2015). A new disease cluster: Mast cell activation syndrome, postural orthostatic tachycardia syndrome, and Ehlers-Danlos syndrome. *Journal of Allergy and Clinical Immunology, 135*(2), AB65.
- Cohen, S. E., Hooper, S. R., Javalkar, K., Haberman, C., Fenton, N., Lai, H., Rutledge, C., Cantu, G., Zhang, D., & Ferris, M. (2015). Self-management and transition readiness assessment: Concurrent, predictive, and discriminant validation of the STARx questionnaire. *Journal of Pediatric Nursing, 30*(5), 668–676.
- College Board. (n.d.). *Accommodations on College Board exams*.
- Dysautonomia International. (2019). *Classroom accommodations for children with dysautonomia*.
- Dysautonomia International. (2023). *Postural orthostatic tachycardia syndrome*.
- Eccles, J. A., Thompson, B., Themelis, K., Amato, M. L., Stocks, R., Pound, A., Jones, C. L., & Harrison, N. A. (2021). Beyond bones: The relevance of variants of connective tissue (hypermobility) to fibromyalgia, ME/CFS and controversies

surrounding diagnostic classification. *Clinical Medicine, 21*(1), 53–58.

- Fu, Q., Vangundy, T. B., Galbreath, M. M., Shibata, S., Jain, M., Hastings, J. L., Bhella, P. S., Levine, J. A., Bundgaard-Nielsen, M., Drummer, C., & Levine, B. D. (2010). Cardiac origins of the postural orthostatic tachycardia syndrome. *Journal of the American College of Cardiology, 55*(25), 2858–2868.
- Garfinkel, S. N., Tiley, C., O'Keeffe, S., Harrison, N. A., Seth, A. K., & Critchley, H. D. (2016). Discrepancies between dimensions of interoception in autism. *Biological Psychology, 114*, 117–126.
- Got Transition. (2020). *Six Core Elements of Health Care Transition 3.0.*
- Herts, K. L., Wallis, E., & Maslow, G. R. (2014). College freshmen with chronic illness: A comparison with healthy first-year students. *Journal of College Student Development, 55*(5), 475–480.
- Huynh, P., Brown, A., Campisi, L., Mruk, A., Nguyen, T., Raschka, M., & Afolabi, T. (2024). Management of postural orthostatic tachycardia syndrome in pediatric patients: A clinical review. *Journal of Pediatric Pharmacology and Therapeutics, 29*(5), 456–467.
- Individuals with Disabilities Education Act, 20 U.S.C. § 1400 et seq. (2004).
- Kizilbash, S. J., Ahrens, S. P., Bruce, B. K., Chelimsky, G., Driscoll, S. W., Harbeck-Weber, C., Mack, K. J., & Fischer, P. R. (2014). Adolescent fatigue, POTS, and recovery: A guide for clinicians. *Current Problems in Pediatric and Adolescent Health Care, 44*(5), 108–133.
- Malfait, F., Francomano, C., Byers, P., Belmont, J., Berglund, B., Black, J., Bloom, L., Bowen, J. M., Brady, A. F., Burrows, N. P., Castori, M., Cohen, H., Colombi, M., Demirdas, S., De Backer, J., De Paepe, A., Fournel-Gigleux, S., Frank, M., Ghali,

N., Giunta, C., Grahame, R., Hakim, A., Jeunemaitre, X., Johnson, D., Juul-Kristensen, B., Kapferer-Seebacher, I., Kazkaz, H., Kosho, T., Lavallee, M.-E., Levy, H., Mendoza-Londono, R., Pepin, M., Pope, F. M., Reinstein, E., Robert, L., Rohrbach, M., Sanders, L., Sobey, G. J., Van Damme, T., Vandersteen, A., van Mourik, C., Voermans, N., Wheeldon, N., Zschocke, J., Tinkle, B., & The International Consortium on the Ehlers-Danlos Syndromes. (2017). The 2017 international classification of the Ehlers-Danlos syndromes. *American Journal of Medical Genetics Part C: Seminars in Medical Genetics, 175*(1), 8–26.

- McManus, M., White, P., Schmidt, A., Barr, M., Langer, C., Barger, K., & Ware, A. (2020). Health care gap affects 20% of United States population: Transition from pediatric to adult health care. *Health Policy OPEN, 1*, 100007.
- National Association of School Nurses. (n.d.). *2022 school nurse workforce data.*
- Pinquart, M., & Shen, Y. (2011). Depressive symptoms in children and adolescents with chronic physical illness: An updated meta-analysis. *Journal of Pediatric Psychology, 36*(4), 375–384.
- Raj, S. R. (2013). Postural tachycardia syndrome (POTS). *Circulation, 127*(23), 2336–2342.
- Raj, S. R., Guzman, J. C., Harvey, P., Richer, L., Schondorf, R., Seifer, C., Thibodeau-Jarry, N., & Sheldon, R. S. (2020). Canadian Cardiovascular Society position statement on postural orthostatic tachycardia syndrome (POTS) and related disorders of chronic orthostatic intolerance. *Canadian Journal of Cardiology, 36*(3), 357–372.
- Roma, M., Marden, C. L., De Wandele, I., Francomano, C. A., & Rowe, P. C. (2018). Postural tachycardia syndrome and other forms of orthostatic intolerance in Ehlers-Danlos syndrome. *Autonomic Neuroscience, 215*, 89–96.

- Sawicki, G. S., Lukens-Bull, K., Yin, X., Demars, N., Huang, I.-C., Livingood, W., Reiss, J., & Wood, D. (2011). Measuring the transition readiness of youth with special healthcare needs: Validation of the TRAQ—Transition Readiness Assessment Questionnaire. *Journal of Pediatric Psychology, 36*(2), 160–171.
- Shaw, B. H., Stiles, L. E., Bourne, K., Green, E. A., Shibao, C. A., Okamoto, L. E., Garland, E. M., Gamboa, A., Diedrich, A., Raj, V., Sheldon, R. S., Biaggioni, I., Robertson, D., & Raj, S. R. (2019). The face of postural tachycardia syndrome: Insights from a large cross-sectional online community-based survey. *Journal of Internal Medicine, 286*(4), 438–448.
- Shibao, C., Arzubiaga, C., Roberts, L. J., II, Raj, S., Black, B., Harris, P., & Biaggioni, I. (2005). Hyperadrenergic postural tachycardia syndrome in mast cell activation disorders. *Hypertension, 45*(3), 385–390.
- Sheldon, R. S., Grubb, B. P., II, Olshansky, B., Shen, W.-K., Calkins, H., Brignole, M., Raj, S. R., Krahn, A. D., Morillo, C. A., Stewart, J. M., Sutton, R., Sandroni, P., Friday, K. J., Hachul, D. T., Cohen, M. I., Lau, D. H., Mayuga, K. A., Moak, J. P., Sandhu, R. K., Kanjwal, K., & Heart Rhythm Society. (2015). 2015 Heart Rhythm Society expert consensus statement on the diagnosis and treatment of postural tachycardia syndrome, inappropriate sinus tachycardia, and vasovagal syncope. *Heart Rhythm, 12*(6), e41–e63.
- Social Security Administration. (2023). *Annual statistical report on the Social Security Disability Insurance program.*
- Tennessee Department of Education. (2023). *Special education and Section 504 services toolkit for school nurses.*
- U.S. Department of Education, Office for Civil Rights. (2011). *Students with disabilities preparing for postsecondary education: Know your rights and responsibilities.*

- U.S. Department of Education, Office for Civil Rights. (2020). *Protecting students with disabilities: Frequently asked questions about Section 504 and the education of children with disabilities.*
- U.S. Department of Education, Office for Civil Rights. (2022). *How to file a discrimination complaint with the Office for Civil Rights.*
- U.S. Department of Health and Human Services. (2025). *Your rights under HIPAA.*
- U.S. Department of Justice. (2006). *A guide to disability rights laws.*
- U.S. Equal Employment Opportunity Commission. (1992). *Your employment rights as an individual with a disability.*
- Valent, P., Akin, C., Bonadonna, P., Hartmann, K., Brockow, K., Castells, M., Escribano, L., Hauswirth, A. W., Kluin-Nelemans, H., Hermine, O., Arock, M., Niedoszytko, M., Schwartz, L. B., Triggiani, M., Shomali, W., Sotlar, K., Sperr, W. R., Kovanen, P. T., Reiter, A., George, T. I., Kristensen, T., Traina, F., Carter, M. C., Metcalfe, D. D., & Akin, C. (2019). Proposed diagnostic algorithm for patients with suspected mast cell activation syndrome. *The Journal of Allergy and Clinical Immunology: In Practice, 7*(4), 1125–1133.
- Younger, J., Parkitny, L., & McLain, D. (2014). The use of low-dose naltrexone (LDN) as a novel anti-inflammatory treatment for chronic pain. *Clinical Rheumatology, 33*(4), 451–459.

Not included because I could not confirm them as cited

- Chopra, P. (2024). *Connecting the dots in EDS, MCAS, POTS, tethered cord syndrome, CCI, Chiari malformation and more. The EDS Clinic.*
- Fegran, L., Hall, E. O. C., Uhrenfeldt, L., Aagaard, H., & Ludvigsen, M. S. (2024). *From pediatrics to adult care: Experiences of transition among youth with a chronic medical*

condition. A meta-ethnography. International Journal of Nursing Studies, 150, 104656.

- Raffaele, L. M. (2024). *Advocating for students with chronic health conditions. Education Law Center.*

Made in United States
Troutdale, OR
10/08/2026

55442342R00100